Essential

Textbook of Medical Jurisprudence

(Forensic Medicine)

By

Izharul H. MD (PSM)

Rajiv Gandhi University, Bangalore

India

CS Independent Publishing Platform, South Carolina, North Charleston, USA

Book Details

Paperback: 299 pages

Publisher: CS Independent Publishing Platform; 1 edition (November 28, 2014)

Language: English

ISBN-10: **1508841934**

ISBN-13: **978-1508841937**

Product Dimensions: 7 x 10 inches

This book has been published in good faith that the material provided by editor/author(s) contained herein is original, and is intended for educational purposes only. Every effort is made to ensure accuracy of material, but publisher and printing platform will not be held responsible for any inadvertent errors, liability, or loss incurred, directly or indirectly, from the use or application of any of the contents of this work. If not specifically stated, all figures and tables are courtesy of the author.

Corresponding email: drizharnium@gmail.com

Contact: 91-8287833547

Essential Textbook of Medical Jurisprudence

First Edition: 2015

Publisher: CS Independent Publishing Platform; 1 edition

Preface to the First Edition

It is indeed a great pleasure to present the first edition of the book **"Essential TextBook of Medical jurisprudence"** with an elegant look. Any individuals, societies, or organizations discussed in this book are mentioned without malice. To the best of my knowledge I am reporting the truth, not with the intent to harm but to inform to the best of my ability as a scholar who has devoted years of research to this significant social theme. The common good requires that such a major hazard to health be given public comment.

First edition of Essential textbook of medical jurisprudence represents a truly remarkable accomplishment within the medical jurisprudence. This book is written, especially for persons in studying and training for board-type examinations, the text is a comprehensive yet concise about medical jurisprudence that actually covers many forensic topics that are largely ignored or only briefly mentioned by many other forensic texts. The book represents an excellent resource for medical jurisprudence/forensic medicine practitioners, forensic pathologists and others within the forensic community.

The entire concept of this book is to give information in as few words as possible without omitting necessary details. Some topics (medical jurisprudence and legal procedures, identification, injuries, sexual offences) which are important point of view are in more details. All topics are updated and recent advances have been incorporated wherever needed.

Essential text book of medical jurisprudence is a teacher friendly book because it meets the long standing desire of teachers for a comprehensive text book that provides a balanced coverage of medical jurisprudence.

This book is student-friendly because it is written in an understandable way, covering the entire syllabus. The matter is presented in such a way as to avoid confusion and to make the reading of the book a pleasurable experience. The lucid language of the book would facilitate quick revision.

It is my hope that this new book will find favorable response from medical students and also offer significant help to medical practitioners, in-service doctors and forensic scientists.

Despite my sincere efforts to make the book accurate and comprehensive as I could, it is possible there may be some gaps or errors in the book. I would be most grateful to the readers specially students and teaching communities, if these deficiencies are pointed out so that can be removed in the next edition. I also invite healthy suggestions from all readers and students to help me improve the quality of book and achieve the purpose with which it has been written. All such feedback would be carefully considered and gratefully acknowledged.

Izharul Hasan

ACKNOWLEDGEMENT

First and foremost, I have to thank my parents for their love and support throughout my life. Thank you both for giving me strength to reach the stars and chase my dreams. My brothers, sisters, and other family members deserve my wholehearted thanks as well.

I would like to express my gratitude to the many people who saw me through this book; to all those who provided support, talked things over, read, wrote, offered comments, allowed me to quote their remarks and assisted in the editing, proofreading and design.

I would like to thank my wife for standing beside me throughout my career and writing this book. She has been my inspiration and motivation for continuing to improve my knowledge and move my career forward.

I would like to thanks my all friends for understanding and encouragement in my many, many moments of crisis. Your friendship makes my life a wonderful experience. I cannot list all the names here, but you are always on my mind.

I wish to express my solemn sentiments and sincere gratitude to all the authors and researches of various textbooks and journal articles which was referred to, while preparing the manuscript of the book without which the scientific base of facts mentioned would not have been possible.

Once again thanks my parents and family members, for sharing my happiness when starting this book and following with encouragement when it seemed too difficult to be completed. I would have probably give up without their support and example on what to do when you really want something.

Last but not least, I wish to offer my apologies to all my colleagues and friends whose name has been omitted inadvertently, for without their constant support, encouragement and well-wishes, the book would not have been completed.

Thank you, Lord, for always being there for me.

Izharul Hasan

Index

Chapter 1

MEDICAL JURISPRUDENCE AND LEGAL PROCEDURE

Forensic or Legal Medicine

Forensic or Legal Medicine (forensic = of or used in courts of law) is defined as the subject dealing with application of medical and paramedical knowledge to solve legal problems which helps in administration of justice, e.g. Medical examination reports of cases of injuries (assault, attempt of murder etc), sexual offences (rape, sodomy etc), poisoning are being considered as evidence by criminal courts to decide whether the accused was guilty of the charge[1].

The purpose of forensic medicine is to introduce the fundamental concepts in these disciplines to police officers, lawyers, medical students, pathologists, residents and physicians. The subject is chosen to cover all of the basic facts of death and related issues commonly witnessed during the medicolegal work. An expert of forensic medicine is one who has amassed his knowledge through experience, common sense and scientific interpretation. The secrets of disease or crime are always hidden in silent soul: The Dead Body[2].

Medical Jurisprudence

Medical Jurisprudence (Juris = law; prudentia = knowledge) deals with legal aspects of medicine, i.e. , medical practice; it also considers legal responsibilities of physician; i.e. examination and treatment of ill or injured or poisoned human subjects lawfully. Such as, medical negligence cases, consent, rights and duties of doctors, infamous conduct, medical ethics etc[1].

Forensic medicine and medical jurisprudence are not synonyms but *interrelated terms.*[1]

State medicine

It is concerned with public, community, and environmental health. It deals with the application of medical to prevent the spread of disease. It is the responsibility of the State to preserve the health of the public. Accordingly, a registered medical practitioner has certain statuary duties: he must inform the public health authorities of

a) Births
b) Deaths
c) Notifiable diseases
d) Cases of food poisoning from a hotel, restaurant, or other eating establishments so that appropriate medical statistics are maintained and spread of disease prevented by suitable measures-quarantine, preventive inoculation, disinfection, control of vectors, etc.[3]

Medical Ethics

Medical ethics deals with the normal principles which should guide members of the medical profession in their dealings with each other, their patients and the state.[1]

Medical Etiquette

Medical etiquette deals with the conventional laws of the courtesy observed between fellow members of the medical profession.[1]

LEGAL PROCEDURES

The Indian legal system was founded by the colonial British by the establishing various courts and enacting statutes for the administration of justice similar to the British Legal System, which was adopted after independence by making some amendments and modification of statutes. The administration of justice in criminal matters are mainly governed by the Indian Penal Code (IPC) 1860, Criminal Procedure Court (CrPC) 1861 and Indian Evidence Act (IEA) 1869, with amendments done on later dates.

Medical officers, in the course of their professional practice, are required to issue medical certificates to their patients for various acts and administrative purpose. They also need to examine the victims and accuse persons involved in various criminal offences and to submit reports, for which the medical officer may be summoned to appear in the court to give evidence in relation to the report submitted by them. Therefore, they must have cleared knowledge about the court of law and legal and criminal procedures.[2]

INDIAN PENAL CODE (1860)

It defines various offence and their punishments admissible under court of law. Jammu and Kashmir have their own penal code, known as Ranbir penal code.[2]

CRIMINAL PROCEDURES CODE (1973)

It defines the procedure of investigations and trial of offences in whole of India, except the state of Jammu and Kashmir. It also deals with various types of courts and their powers.[2]

INDIAN EVIDENCE ACT (1872)

It relates to evidences, based on which courts come to the conclusion of the case.[2]

INQUEST

An inquest is an inquiry into the cause of death in case of sudden, suspicious and unnatural deaths.

It is required in cases of:

i.   Sudden death in an apparently normal individual.
ii.   All suspected cases of homicides, suicide and accidents, irrespective of the nature of causation.
iii. Vehicular accidents.
iv.   Poisonings.
v.   Deaths under anesthesia, over operation table or alleged caese of medical negligence.
vi.   Dowry related deaths.
vii. Deaths under police custody or police firing.
viii. In all cases where a doctor is not in a position to issue the medical certificate into cause of death (MCCD), viz. in mass disasters, etc.

In these conditions, a doctor must not issue the cause of death certificate and police must be informed regarding the case.[2]

Types of inquest

Four types of inquest are followed:

a) Coroner's inquest
b) Police inquest
c) Magistrate inquest
d) Medical examiner system (in USA)

NOTE: *only police inquest and magistrate inquest are followed in India nowadays[2].*

CORONER

- A coroner is a special officer appointed by government under Coroner's Act, 1871.[2]

- Usually a lawyer is appointed as coroner.[2]

- His rank corresponds to that of first class magistrate.[1,2,3,5]

- In India, only Bombay possesses a coroner.[1,2,3,5]

- He can hold an inquiry into all unnatural and suspicious deaths occurring in his jurisdiction.[2]

POWERS OF CORONER

- To hold inquest in cases of unnatural, accidental or sudden deaths from suspicious or unknown cause.[1,2]

- To hold an inquiry if death occurs in jail or in court of law or in certified schools.[1]

- He can order any medical men to hold post mortem examination.[1]

- He can summon the medical men who attended the case to give evidence.[2]

- He can order for identification of dead body.[1]

- He can appoint a deputy coroner during his sickness or unavoidable absence. (special power).[3]

Difference between coroner's court and magistrate's court

CORONER'S COURT	MAGISTRATE'S COURT
It is a court of inquiry only.	It is a court of trial.
The accused need not to be present during trial.	The accused must be present during the trial.
Coroner has no power to impose fine or award punishment to the accused.	The magistrate can impose fine or punish the accused.

Police Inquest

It is practiced all over India. It is conducted by an officer- in-charge (OC) of a police station or some other police officer empowered by the State government (Section 174 CrPC). The police officer who investigates the case is known as the investigating officer (IO).[2]

- Inquiry should be held by police in all unnatural or suspicious death due to foul play.[3]
- Not below the rank of head constable.[1]
- The Police officer (sub inspector) making the preliminary inquiry is called the " Investigating officer" (I.O.)[1,2,3,5]

- He conducts the inquiry at the site of death with two witness of the area. (panchas or panchayatdars).[1,3]
- He prepares the inquest report known as panchnama or surothal.[3]
- Three copies are prepared; two copies are sent to doctors for Medico legal Autopsy and one copy to the concerned magistrate.[1]

The police officer by writing may order any person, who appears to know about the facts, to answer questions for investigation purpose (section 175 CrPC). The person so ordered is bound to appear before the police officer and answer the questions put to him, otherwise he will be liable under section 179 IPC for not answering the questions.

The police officer may also request the medical officer conducting the postmortem examination to preserve garments, articles or visceras of the dead body for chemical tests or may request to perform such tests as may be essential for investigation of the case.[2]

Difference between coroner's inquest and police inquest

CORONER'S INQUEST	POLICE INQUEST
1. Inquest held by coroner who is highly qualified and experienced and thus superior to police inquest	1. Inquest held by police officer who is not qualified either in law and medicine.
2. Held only in Bombay.	2. Held all over India except Bombay.
3. He is not required to inform magistrate about the crime.	3. He has to inform the magistrate.
4. Witnesses do not sign the inquest report.	4. Panchayatdars or witnesses have to sign the report.
5. He can issue warrant for the arrest of accused.	5. He cannot issue warrant but can arrest an accused in cognizable offence.
6. He can summon the doctor to give evidence.	6. He cannot summon the doctor to give evidence.
7. He can order the body to be exhumed.	7. He cannot order exhumation.[1]

Magistrate's Inquest

In some conditions, the police are not authorized to hold inquest. It is then conducted by an executive magistrate or any other magistrate specifically authorized by state government for this purpose (section 176 CrPC).[2]

- It is Conducted by a Magistrate of first class or an executive magistrate.[1,2,3,5]
- It is made in cases of:-

1) Deaths in prison. [1,2,3,5]

2) Deaths in police custody. [1,2,3,5]

3) Deaths due to police firing, lathi charge and other actions. [1,2,3,5]

4) Exhumation. [1,2,3,5]

5) Death of bride within seven years of her marriage and dowry death under section 304 B of the IPC.[1,2,3,5]

6) Deaths in psychiatric hospital.[2]

7) Death in borstal school or reformatories.[2]

In some cases of great public interest, a magistrate can hold inquest instead of or in addition to a police inquest.[2]

Reasons of Magistrate's Inquest
- No person is deprived of his liberty and his rights as a citizen.
- No person is allowed to die, deprived of his right due to neglect or brutality by the people in whose charge he/she is.
- Doubt about the identity, cause of death, or manner of death of a person.[4]

Medical Examiner's system

This system is practiced in some states of the US. In this system, doctors having qualification in pathology and forensic medicine are appointed as medical examiners. The medical examiners visit the scene of crime, prepare the inquest report and also conduct the postmortem examination. As the inquest reports and post mortem examination reports are prepared by the same medical examiner, it is far superior to the other systems of inquest, but the medical examiner does not have any judicial powers. *This type of inquest is not held in India.*

- Prevalent in the USA
- Forensic pathologist

- It has no judicial function similar to the coroner or judicial magistrate
- Superior to all other types of inquest[3]

Courts

- In India there are two kinds of court :

1. Criminal court.

2. Civil court.[1,2,3,5]

Civil courts

Civil courts deal with the civil matters- mainly disputes between two or more parties under provision of the civil procedure code and Indian Evidence Act relating to land and property, administrative, industrial, labor, financial and family matters. Civil courts do not award punishments, but decide the cases in favor of one or more parties on the basis of facts produced before it or award monetary compensation to an aggrieved party. Motor accidents claim tribunals, industrial tribunals, labor and family courts are civil courts function under specific Acts for limited purposes.[2]

Criminal courts of India

Criminal courts try the various offences codified in the Indian Penal Code and award punishment or acquit the accused person after detailed trial proceedings. The procedure of trial, recording evidence and awarding punishments are guided by the provisions of Indian Evidence Act, Code of Criminal Procedures and Indian Penal Code.[2]

The criminal courts are of four types:

➤ Supreme Court

➤ High Courts

➤ Session Courts

➤ Magistrate's Courts[1,2,3,5]

Supreme Court

- Also called Apex court or Appellate court.[7]
- Established on 28 January 1950.[7]
- It is highest court established at New Delhi, which does not take any case *prima facie* (At first appearance).[7]
- Instituted by *Part V, Chapter IV* of the Indian Constitution.[7]

- *Articles 124 – 147* of the Constitution of India lay down the composition and jurisdiction of the Supreme Court. [7]
- The judgments and decisions declare by it are binding on all courts in India. [2]
- After hearing the appellant and the opposite sides, it can enhance or reduce the quantum of punishments awarded by the lower courts or acquit the convict of charges made against him. [2]
- It only takes cases referred from state High courts. [1,3]
- But a person can approach Apex court in case of violation of his / her fundamental rights under *article 32 of the constitution.* [7]

High Court

- High courts are the highest judicial tribunal in a state and established mostly in the state capitals except Uttarpradesh. [1]
- Currently 24 High Courts at state and Union Territory level. [7]
- High Courts are instituted as constitutional courts under article 214 of the Indian Constitution. [7]
- It only takes cases referred from session courts. [1,3]
- But a person can approach the High court in case of violation of his / her fundamental rights under article 266 of the constitution. [7]
- A death sentence awarded by a court of session judge has to be confirmed by a division bench of the High Court. [2]
- High Courts have the power to award any sentence authorized by law and can upheld, enhance or reduce the quantum of punishment awarded by session courts on an appeal or acquit the convict. If not satisfied, the convict can appeal before the Supreme Court against the judgment of High Court. [2]

District Court / Session court

- These are established in the District headquarters and Metropolitan cities. [1,2,3,5]
- They can only try cases referred to them by First Class Magistrate or Assistant session judges. [1,3]
- A session court is headed by a sessions judge, who supervises the functions of the different judicial courts in the district. He allocates cases to other judges, which are commited to the sessions court for trial by the magistrates. [1,2]
- A session judge and additional session judges have same judicial powers. They can pass any sentence authorized by law, including a death sentence passed by a session court must be confirmed by the High Court. [2]

- An assistant session judge can pass any sentence authorized by law, except death sentence, life imprisonment or imprisonment exceeding 10 years. He can pass unlimited amount of fine.[2]

Magistrate's Court

Judicial magistrates are of three types:

(a) **Chief judicial or chief Metropolitan Court,**

(b) **First class judicial magistrate's court or Metropolitan Magistrate's Court.**

(c) **Second class Magistrate's Court.**[1,2,3,5]

In Metropolitan cities, the Chief judicial magistrate and first class judicial magistrate are designated as Chief Metropolitan Magistrate (CMM) and Metropolitan Magistrate(MM) respectively.[2]

(a) **Chief judicial or Chief Metropolitan Court:** In each district, there is a Chief Judicial Magistrate who is, in general, control of all other judicial magistrates in the district. He commutes all session's triable cases of the session court for trial. A chief judicial magistrate can pass a sentence of imprisonment up to 7 years and unlimited amount of fine.[2]

(b) **First class judicial magistrate's court or Metropolitan Magistrate's Court:** can pass sentence of imprisonment up to 3 years and fine up to Rs. 10,000/- or both.[2]

(c) **Second class Magistrate's Court:** can pass a sentence of imprisonment not exceeding 1 year and fine up to Rs. 5000/- or both.[3]

All the judicial magistrates can pass through both the sentences (imprisonment and fine) together.[2]

Powers of judges and magistrates

JUDGE/ MAGISTRATE	DEATH SENTENCE	IMPRISONMENT	SOLITARY CONFINEMENT	FINE
SUPREME COURT JUDGE	Upheld / confirm	Yes – any number of years.	Yes	Any amount.

HIGH COURT JUDGE	Upheld / confirm	Do	Yes	yes
DISTRICT & CITY SESSION JUDGE	Yes (but to be confirmed by High court)	Do	Yes	yes
ASSISTANT SESSION JUDGE	No	Up to 10 years	Yes	yes
CHIEF JUDICIAL/ METROPO LITAN MAGISTRA TE	No	Up to 7 years	Yes	yes
FIRST CLASS JUDICIAL MAGISTRA TE	No	Up to 3 years	Yes	Rs 10,000 (after 2005 amendment act)
SECOND CLASS JUDICIAL MAGISTRA TE	No	Up to 1 year	Yes	Rs 5000 (after 2005 amendment act

Punishments Authorized by Law in India

The punishments are provided under section 53 of IPC.[4]

1. **Death sentence or Capital punishment:** It is passed by the court of session judge , which is to be confirmed by the High Court. It is awarded in cases of murder, rape with murder, murder committed by a life convict, dacoity with murder, waging war against Government of India and repeated offences under the Narcotic Drugs and Psychotropic substances.

   In India death sentence is carried out by hanging, commonly known as judicial hanging. Other methods used to execute a convict in some other countries are: electrocution, firing by firing squad, gas chamber, guillotine, injection of lethal dose of some sedatives drugs and poisons.[2,4]

2. **Life imprisonment- Review after 14 years, if no bad record then released:** it is also awarded by the Court of Session judge. Usually, it comprises imprisonment for 20 years, which can be reduced to 14 years for good behavior by the imprisonment. At present, the life imprisonment is for the rest of life of the convict. [2,4]

3. **Imprisonment** – it is of two types:

- **Rigorous imprisonment:** means imprisonment without hard labor.

- **Simple imprisonment including solitary confinement:** it is imprisonment with hard labor. The prisoner is to work in the prison according to his skill and physical ability. A prisoner may be ordered to pass a part of his period of rigorous imprisonment in solitary confinement. [2,4]

4. **Forfeiture of property:** court can order attachment of both movable and immovable property of a person. [2,4]

5. **Fine:** court can impose monetary fine only or in addition to imprisonment in some cases. [2,4]

6. **Treatment, training and rehabilitation:** court may order detention of juvenile offender found guilty of a crime in a borstal school or reformatories till completion of 18 years of age. [2,4]

Note: - whipping and transportation (kala paani) has now abolished.[4]

Proceedings in Court

* Summons

* Subpoena

* Oath of Affirmation

* Recording of evidence / Proof

* Decision of Judge / Court

* Execution of Court orders[1,2]

Summons

It is a written order issued by a court to a witness compelling his attendance in the court on a specific date, time and place to give evidence under penalty (section 61 to 69 of CrPC). It is issued in duplicate, signed by the presiding officer of the court. It also bears the seal of the court. The name of the accused person and the case number and the sections of IPC under which the person is to be prosecuted are also mentioned.[2]

- It is a command or order issued by a court to an accused person or witness, whose attendance is required in the court.[1]

- It must be written in duplicate, signed and sealed by presiding officer of the court.[1]

Subpoena *(sub- under, poena- penalty)*

- It is a document compelling the attendence of witness in the court under penalty.[1]

- Witness is to attend court in specified date and hour and Produce documents, if asked for and give evidence.[1]

- Non-compliance to summons in a civil case may render one liable to action for damages, i.e. fine, but in a criminal case, fine or even imprisonment may be ordered. He cannot leave the court without the permission of the magistrate or the judge after evidence. If he fails to attend in time, warrant can be issue to compel his attendance.[2]

Cases on the same day?

If the medical officer is to attend two courts- one civil and another criminal on a particular day, criminal case would get preference over the civil cases. Criminal cases of higher courts get the preference over the lower court summons. Medical officer must inform the other court which he is not attending with reasons. In case of same ranking courts, summons received earliest will have to attend first.[2]

- Criminal courts have precedence over civil court
- Criminal cases of higher courts gets preference over lower courts
- The court which served the summons first receives preference[1]

Failure to obey Summons

- *Civil case-* pay damages i.e. fine.
- *Criminal case-* fine or imprisonment / warrant of arrest may be ordered.[1]

Conduct money

- *In civil cases*- Medical officer gets a fee to cover the expenses incurred towards attending the civil court. Usually, this is paid when a summon is served to doctor. If not paid, then doctor can bring it to the notice of the magistrate/ judge.
- *In criminal cases*- where state is the prosecuting party, Government medical officer will not get any fee but he is paid the travelling allowances. In private criminal cases, government medical officers will get fee. Private practitioners get fees either from the court or from the private parties concerned, when ordered as such by the court.[1,3]

Witness

A witness is a person who gives a statement or testimony under oath or solemn affirmation in the court of law. All persons are competent to give evidence unless they are incapable of understanding the questions put to them or giving rational answer to these questions, due to tender year, extreme old age or disease.[2]

Types of witness

There are two types of witness:

- Common witness
- Expert or skilled[3]

1. *Common witness:* is that person who narrates what he has heard or perceived or states the facts observed by himself. He is not able to draw any inference from observations made by him or express any option from observations made by other.[1,3]

2. *Expert witness:* on account of his professional training and skills, is capable of giving opinion observed by himself. e.g. Medical men, Chemical examiners, thumb and fingerprint expert, handwriting expert.[1,3]

   To be an expert medical witness, a person having recognized medical degree must be registered with any of the state medical council. The Indian Medical Council Act, 1956, in section 15 (2) (b), states no person other than a medical practitioner enrolled on a state medical register shall be entitled to give evidence at any inquest or in any court of law as an expert under section 45 of the Indian Evidence Act 1872 on any matter relating to medicine.[2]

   - *A medical man is both common and expert witness. Common because he can say the size, position and number of wounds; Expert because he can say whether the wound is ante-mortem or post-mortem, accidental, homicidal or suicidal, age of wounds.*[1,2,3,5]

- **Hostile witness:-** is one who suppresses facts or who gives half truth or who gives false evidence. Hostile witness is a witness who deliberately gives false evidence in the court of law either by concealing a part or whole of the truth or making totally false statement, which he knows to be false or not true and thereby contradicts his previous statements made before the same court or in a previous statements made before the same court or in a previous judicial proceeding (section 191 IPC). Court may declare a witness hostile when suggested by the lawyer of the party who summoned the witness. Leading questions can be asked to a hostile witness during examination in chief.[2]

- **Skilled or scientific witness:-** are also called expert witnesses they have specialized knowledge of technical subjects.

EVIDENCE

It is the deposition of a witness in the court of law, under oath, relating to a particular fact in issue, recorded and accepted by the court. Under section 3 of Indian Evidence Act, Evidence is defined as what a court of justice is permitted by law to take into consideration for making clear or ascertaining the the truth of the fact or point in issue. Thus evidence means and includes:

1. All statements, which the court permits or requires to be made before it by witness in relation to matters of fact under inquiry. Such statements are called oral evidence.
2. All documents including electronic records produced for inspection of the court. Such documents are called documentary statement.[2]

Forms of evidence

There may be 4 forms:

1. Oral

2. Documentary

3. Direct or evidence of eyewitness

4. Indirect or circumstantial or hearsay[1]

Oral evidence

All statements which the court permits or requires to be made before it by witnesses in relation to the fact under enquiry.[2]

- It is defined by section 3 of The Indian Evidence Act.[4]

  It is something which the witness has seen, heard or perceived personally.[4]

- It is superior to documentary evidence since the person has to prove on oath that the evidence is true and is crossly examined.[1,2,3,4,5]

- Section 60 of The Indian Evidence Act states that oral evidence must be direct means- who says he saw it and who heard he saw it.[4]

Documentary evidence

- It means all documents produced for inspection of the court.[1,2]

- Documents mean any matter expressed or described upon any substance by means of letters, figures or marks, which may be used for the purpose of recording that matter (section 29 IPC).[2]

- They are:

i. Medical certificate of ill health and insanity.

ii. Medical certificate of death.

iii. Medico legal reports : injury report, postmortem report, rape, abortion, poisoning, drunkenness certificate etc.[1,3]

Documents can be proved either by primary evidence or secondary evidence (section 61 IEA):

Primary evidence:- when the original document is produced in the court for inspection (section 62 IEA).[2]

Secondary evidence:- when the certified copies, duplicate copies or copies made from the original by mechanical process or copies made from the original are produced in the court (section 63 IEA).[2]

Direct evidence

- It is the evidence of what the witness has personally seen or gathered from his senses.

- Also includes production of an original document.[1]

Indirect evidence

- The witness here presents what was told to him by third party.

- Also called hearsay evidence.

- Has no legal value.[1]

Hearsay Evidence

It is the evidence given by person who had no direct knowledge regarding the incident (fact in issue), but came to know about it from somebody who had seen, heard or perceived the matter directly.[1,3]

Dying Declarations

- Section 32 (1) of Indian Evidence act describes dying declaration.[4]
- It is a statement verbal or written made by a person who had died explaining the cause and circumstances of his death.[4]
- It is based on legal maxim *'nemo moriturus praesumitur mentire* 'i.e. a man will not meet his Maker with a lie in his mouth.[4]
- This is admitted as documentary evidence but if the person survives then it has no legal value as dying declaration.[1,3,4]

PROCEDURE

- When a severely injured person is brought to hospital, the MO informs the magistrate through local PS to have dying declaration recorded.
- If the patient is critical and magistrate will take time to arrive then MO himself can record dying declaration in presence of two witnesses.
- Usually recorded in forms of questions and answers without any prompting.
- Should be recorded in patient's own vernacular.
- No suggestions or leading questions allowed.
- No outsider is allowed.
- After completion, it should be read over to the patient.
- Should be signed by him or thumb impression is inserted.
- If a doctor record's it, it is also signed by witness.
- Then it is sent to court through local PS in a sealed envelope marked 'dying declaration'.[1]

Dying deposition

- It is a statement made by a dying person under oath and recorded by magistrate in the presence of the accused or his lawyer, who is allowed to cross examine the person. As oath is administered, it is like a bed side court.[2]
- It is always recorded by the Magistrate.

- Accused or his lawyer must be present.
- It is more valuable than dying declaration as the accused has got opportunity to challenge and cross-examined.
- The Medical Officer's presence is necessary to certify the mental fitness of the patient (compos mentis).[1]

Difference between dying declaration and dying deposition

Dying Declaration	Dying Deposition
It may be recorded by a medical Officer.	It is recorded only by the Magistrate.
Oath is not necessary.	Oath is necessary.
Presence of accused or his lawyer is not required.	Accused or his lawyer may be present.
Cross examination is not possible.	Cross examination is permitted.
Legal value is less (as accused or his lawyer not present).	Legal value is more (as it is almost a bed side court).

Procedure of Recording of Evidence[1]

- Oath taking
- Examination-in-chief
- Cross-examination
- Re-examination by public prosecutor
- Questions put up by Judge/Magistrate

Oath-taking

- Before deposition starts, witness must take oath.[1]
- Unoathed evidence is not admissible to the court of law, except when a person is below 7 years of age or when he is mentally deranged-both cannot understand the importance of taking oath but they may depose when they speak the truth.[2]
- Oath is as follows: "I solemnly affirm that I shall give the truth, nothing but the truth and I conceal nothing, if anything given false, so help me God."[1]

- The witness may be prosecuted for *perjury* (misguiding the court) under section 193 of I.P.C.[4]

Examination-in-chief

- This is done by the prosecution side i.e. by the public prosecutor or the lawyer who calls the witness.[1]
- In this stage, questions are put to the witness and answers elicited and recorded by the court.[2]
- No leading questions are allowed. (leading questions are one which suggest their own answers.)[1]
- Leading questions are those which suggest their own answers or the answered wish for or answered as 'yes' or 'no', e.g. did you see Mr. K. hit Mr. Y. by an iron rod? IT should be- where had you been in such time? What did you see? With what object did he hit?[1]
- Here, witness has to relate the facts fully within his knowledge regarding the case. But if the judge is convinced that the witness is hostile, leading questions may be allowed by him to re-examine the witness by public prosecutor.[2]
- It is described under section 137 of Indian Evidence Act.[4]

Cross Examination

- This is made by the lawyer of opposite party i.e. defense lawyer.[1]
- He will try to weaken the evidence given by the witness in the examination in chief.[1]
- He will try to prove before the court that the evidence is untrustworthy and unbelievable.[1]
- In this stage, leading questions are allowed.[1]
- There is no time limit for cross examination. It may last for hours or even days. Of course the judge or the magistrate may disallow irrelevant questions and cut short the cross examination.[1]

Re-examination

- This is done by the prosecution side, in order to clear up certain ambiguities or discrepancies that might have been made by the witness in the cross examination.[1]
- To remove any doubts that may have arisen during cross examination.[1]
- Leading questions are not allowed.[1]
- No questions related to new matters, are to be asked (without the permission of the court). If new matters are asked, the defense will take another chance of cross examination.[1]

Court Questions

- The judge or magistrate can ask question to witness at any stage to clarify some points.[3]
- He can call witness again for his evidence, if needed by the court, related to the same case[3].
- The courts also have power to recall and re-examine any witness already examined, if it appears to the court that re-examination of the witness is essential to clear some points before taking any decision in the case (section 165 IEA and section 311 CrPC).[2]

Warrant

- It is a written order- sign & seal of presiding officer of court.[2]
- It should bear name & designation of person who is to execute it.[2]
- It Indicates name & address of accused.[2]
- It must state the offence he is accused of.[2]
- It should indicate date of issue.[2]

OFFENCE

Offence is an act of commission or omission made punishable by any law (section 40 IPC and section 2 (n) CrPC).[2]

TYPES OF OFFENCE

Offences are of two types:

a. Non-cognizable offence
b. Cognizable offece[2]

Non-Cognizable offence

- Any offence for which the police officer cannot arrest the accused without a warrant
- E.g. Bribery, defamation, perjury, causing simple hurt, buying/ selling person for slavery[2]

Cognizable offence

- Any offence for which the police officer may arrest the accused without a warrant
- waging war against government, counterfeiting Indian currency, adulteration of food, destroying, damaging or defiling place of worship, theft, robbery, murder, kidnapping, rape, attempting suicide, causing grievous hurt, dowry death, rioting.[2]

Doctor in the Witness box:

Duties of doctor in the witness box are:

i. After receiving the summon, the doctor must attend the court and should be punctual.
ii. He must be well dressed, looking modest and sober.
iii. He should carry along with him, all the records relevant to the case.
iv. Be well prepared about the case.
v. Never discuss the case with anyone outside the court.
vi. Never lose temper in the court.
vii. Should never be nervous inside the court. He should remain calm, polite and courteous.
viii. He should never be over confident.
ix. Avoid using technical terms and always try to explain the case in simple language.
x. If a lawyer quotes the paragraph of a book. He should be asked to show the book or some chapter.
xi. Listen to questions carefully. If it is not audible or not clear, one must ask the lawyer to repeat the question.
xii. Always address the judge by "sir" or "your honor" giving him his due respect.
xiii. He has to answer all the questions and does not have any professional privilege.
xiv. Limit his answer to the expertise in his field and must not volunteer any information or answer questions asked to him beyond his expertise.
xv. After conclusion of his evidence, he should read the written deposition of his evidence recorded by the court and he should put his signature on each page, getting any corrections, if needed, done by the court under his initials. He should not leave the court until he is permitted to leave.

At the end, we can say, as the doctor is said to be a responsible and respectable person of a society, while in the court he should be well dressed, modest, polite and courteous, while giving evidence, to keep the dignity of these professions[2].

Volunteering statement

It is the statement which is made by a witness (MO) without being asked by court during the course of trial with a view to find out the truth. A witness is not supposed to volunteer his statement in a court, unless called for to do so. This may be true, when witness is a lay man, but not always in case of a medical witness. Though a medical witness is called upon by one side to give evidence in the court, he must not forget that he is man of science about honesty and fair dealings, his duties to the opposite party. He must remember that he must help the court with his special knowledge to elicit the truth. Hence, as a scientific expert he thinks the court should be apprised of some facts which have not been asked to him, he should volunteer his statements. [1,7]

REFERANCE

1. Basu S.C. , Hand Book Of Forensic Medicine and Toxicology, *third edition (2007),* Current Distributors, Lenin Saranee, Calcutta.(page no. 1, 3 to 10).
2. Mahanta Putul, Modern Textbook of Forensic Medicine And Toxicology *(2014),* Jaypee Brothers Medical Publishers, Darya Ganj, New Delhi. (Page no. 8 to 13, 16,17,20).
3. Parikh C.K., Parikh's textbook of medical jurisprudence forensic medicine and toxicology, *sixth edition (2011),*C.B.S. Publishers and Distributors, Ansari Road, Darya Ganj, New Delhi. (Page no. 1.3, 1.4, 1.9, 1.17, 1.19).
4. Kumar Avinash, Law Of Evidence, *third edition (2011),* Singhal Law Publications, Burari, Delhi -84. (Page no. 105, 106, 130, 172, 176, 177, 178, 209, 216).
5. Modi. Jaising. P, Textbook of Medical Jurisprudence And Toxicology, Twenty *First Edition (1997),* N.M. Tripathi Private Limited, Bombay.
6. Usmani Hammad, Tib-Ul-Qanoon, *First edition (1976),* Universal Book House, Allahabad. (Page no. 17 to 33).
7. Krishan Vij Textbook of Forensic medicine and Toxicology, 4th Edt.

Chapter 2

IDENTIFICATION

Identification

Identification means fixing the exact personality of an individual. It is the determination of the individuality of a person based on certain physical characteristics. Identification of the person is usually carried out by the police. However, a medical person, in certain situations, has to confirm the identity of an individual based on his medical knowledge. It is done in a living person or dead by recognizing certain specific features that are unique to that person[1].

Identification of a person or dead body means the recognition of that person or dead body. It is based on certain physical characteristics unique to that individual.[2, 5]

By identity is meant the determination of the individuality of a person.[3, 6]

The examination of a person for the purpose of identification should not be not be undertaken without obtaining his free consent, and at the same time it should be explained to him that the facts noted might go in evidence against him.[3]

Types of identification

Identification may be of two types:
1. Complete identification
2. Incomplete identification or partial identification
   - Complete (absolute) identification refers when all the features of a person are known and we can fix the individuality of a person absolutely.
   - Incomplete (partial) identification means when only certain features of an individual are known. (e.g., race sex, age, stature, etc.)[1,2]

Medico-legal circumstances where identification is required

The methods of identification vary with:
   i.   Circumstances of death
   ii.   Time elapsed since death
   iii. Ante-mortem data available for comparison.

Identification may become difficult in case of fire, explosions, advanced decomposition mutilation, mass disasters like earthquakes, aircraft accidents (fig 1), etc. Medico-legal circumstances where identification is required are as narrated in table no.1

Table 1: Medicolegal circumstances where identification is required[1]

1. With living person

Medical purposes	Civil purposes	Criminal purposes
Unconscious patient	Problems of inheritance	Sexual offences
Patient with true amnesia	Marriage	Kidnaping
Mental confusion	Employment or immigration	Determine the criminal personality
	Call for military service	Criminal abortion
	Disputed paternity or maternity	Accused of criminal offences
	Pension, life insurance, voting right	
	Disputed sex	
	Missing person, etc.	

2. With dead person

A missing and presumed dead person
Issuing death certificate
Accused in criminal offences
Mass disaster
Exhumation, etc.

CORPUS DELICTI (THE ESSENCE OF CRIME)

It means the facts of any criminal offence or the body of the crime. The main part of corpus delicti is the establishment of identity of the person, in a case of murder. The corpus delicti includes the body of the victim and other facts, which

31

are indications of foul play like a bullet or apart of the knife found in the body and responsible for death. Photograph of the person depicting injuries, cloths with defects or blood stain and scratches are all included in this. It becomes difficult for the police to solve the crime if the identity of the victim is not known. The identification of the dead body and proof of corpus delicti is essential before a sentence is passed in a murder trial, because to support the false charge, unclaimed decomposed bodies or parts of the bodies may be produced.[1]

The corpus delicti means body of the offence (essence of crime) not the physical body of the victim) and in case of homicide, it includes

- Positive identification of the body,
- Proof of its death by a criminal act of the accused.

Once the identity is established, a trial for murder can take place[2, 3, 6]

POINTS TO BE NOTED FOR THE PURPOSE OF IDENTIFICATION
Commonly recorded data for both living and dead

1. Name (in full)
2. Name of father, family members, relatives
3. Address for correspondence[1]
4. General appearance: weight, height skin color and hair(color, texture, pattern)[1,3]
5. Features: face, eyebrows, iris, chin, nose, configuration of ear, portrait parle, etc.
6. Clothing: Refer the occupation and social status[1]
7. Age
8. Sex [1, 2, 3, 5, 6]
9. Blood group (A,B,AB,O)[1]
10. Prints: fingerprints, footprints, lip prints [1,3, 5, 6]
11. Congenital abnormality: asymmetry, harelip, cleft palate, polydactyl, etc.[1]
12. Birthmarks
13. Occupational marks
14. Scars and moles
15. Tattoos
16. Photographs[1,2,3,5,6]
17. Anthropometry not used nowadays: span of outstretched hands, chest circumference, length of foot, forearm, fingers; ear measurements, shape of the chin or nose etc. [1,2]
18. Race (Negros, Caucasians, Mongoloids)[1, 5, 6]

Methods of identification of living person

1. Personal characters: voice, speech, mental power, education, occupation, handwriting, gait, etc.[1,3]
2. Signature or thumb impression.[1]
3. Identification marks (two).[1,2]
4. Nationality: country of birth.
5. Religion and caste.[1]

Methods of identification of dead person

1) Documents: personal papers, photographs, ID cards, credit cards, etc.
2) Jewelry: rings, bracelets, earrings, watches, lighters, pens, keys.[1,2,3]
3) Contacts traces: give occupational data, e.g. paint, grease, flour, dyes.
4) Height: from the skeleton.
5) Teeth examination
6) Internal physical examination and medical appliances:
   a) underlying disease,
   b) X-ray of the whole body may reveal the old fracture prosthesis like plates or nail, etc.
   c) Pacemakers and
   d) Artificial valve.[1]

7) data from the skull (if previous X-ray is available):
   a) Frontal sinus,
   b) Skull suture pattern and
   c) Vasculature grooves in the skull.[1]
8) The time that the body or bones have been buried.[1]

Identification based on advanced laboratory test

- DNA profile or DNA fingerprinting
- Video graph
- Voice identification
- Superimposition technique
- Facial reconstruction technique
- Digital signature
- Retina and iris scan[1]
- **X-Rays:** age, sex, race, occupation, diagnosis of certain conditions, identification and cause of death.
- **UV-Rays:** use to locate and define tattoo marks and scars on burned and decomposed remains, to interpret illegible ink markings on clothes, and segregate bones in case of mix-up. To see washed blood stains and seminal stains show bluish white fluorescence.

- **Postmortem serology:** a known postmortem boold grouping of an individual serves to narrow the range of possible identities. Congested tissues such as lung, liver or skeletal muscle, putrefied bodies, blood group antigens, bone marrow in skeletal remains can be utilized. [2]

Identification: special techniques

- Dactylography (fingerprints)
- Poroscopy (study of pores)
- Footprints or foot-marks (podogram)
- Cheiloscopy (lip prints)
- Rugoscopy (palatal rugae prints).

DETERMINATION OF RACE

Race can be determined by:

1. **COMPLEXION:** it is of little value. Generally, the skin is brown in Indians, fair in Europeans and black in Negroes. Color of skin is changed in burns and when the body is decomposed.
2. **EYE COLOR:** this is also unreliable. Usually, Indians have black eyes and few have brown eyes. Europeans have blue or gray eyes and Negroes have black eyes.
3. **HAIR:** generally speaking Indians have black thin hair. Europeans have fair or light brown hair. Negroes have their hair arranged in spirals.
4. **CLOTHING:** identifying the race by clothes can be misleading due to changes in the cultural trends.
5. **LIPS:** Black have thick lips that are slightly everted.[2]
6. **TEETH:** The incisors, as well, differ in their basic shape. The incisors fall into two basic shape. The incisors fall into two basic categories, based on the shape of the lingual (tongue) surface of the tooth. These two categories are: shovel-shaped and spatulate or spatula-shaped
   As there is more than one race with spatulate incisors, other indicators are necessary to positively identify race, although this single feature can be used to eliminate one of the possibilities. Each of the following three races has their own shaped incisor, African and European have spatulate, and Asian has shovel-shaped incisor.
7. Skeletal features and indices.
8. Genetic DNA identification will revolutionize this aspect in near future.
9. **PHYSICAL FEATURES:** various physical features of the skull like shape of the orbit, shape of the nasal aperture, and shape of the hard palate are also useful to determine the race. (Table:2)

Table: 2 differentiating points between races from physical features[1]

Features	Caucasian	Mongolian	Negro
Complexion	Fair	Yellowish	Black
Eyes: iris color	Gray or blue	Black	Black
Skull	Rounded with raised forehead	Square, forehead inclined backward	Narrow and elongated with small compressed forehead
Orbit	Triangular	Rounded	Square
Nasal aperture	Elongated	Rounded	Broad
Nose	Sharp	Flattened	Blunt
Face	Small	Large and flattened	Protruding jaw, prominent molar bone with oblique teeth set
Hair palate	Triangular	Rounded	Rectangular
Upper limbs	Proportionate to body	Smaller than trunk	Larger than trunk, forearm larger in comparison to arm, small head
Lower limbs	Proportionate to body	Smaller than trunk	Leg larger in comparison to thigh, feet wide and flat, heel bone projecting backward

The cephalic index: the important test for determining race is the cephalic index or index of breadth, which is obtained by multiplying the maximum breadth of the skull measured transversely by 100 and dividing the result by the greatest length measured from before backwards, skull having the cephalic index between 70 and 74.9, as observed among the aborigines and pure Aryans, are called **mesati-cephalic** and are characteristics of the European and Chinese, while skulls with 80 to 89.9 cephalic index are termed **brachy cephalic** or short headed, as observed in the Mongolian race.[3]

RELIGION AND CASTE

HINDU MALES are not circumcised. Other features like cast marks on the forehead, sacred thread, necklace of wooden beads and tufts of hair on the back of head if present is useful to ascertain the religion.

HINDU FEMALES may have vermilion on the head and forehead, silver toe ornaments, MangalSutra, tattoo marks, nose ring in left nostril with few openings for ear rings along the helix.

MUSLIM FEMALES may have a nose ring aperture in the septum, several openings in the ears along the helix and usually no tattoo marks are found.

MUSLIM MALES are circumcised and callosities may be found on the forehead, knee and ankle due to special attitude adopted during the prayers.[1]

PARSI MALES wear a sacred (kaohti) round the waist and sadra (muslin kurta) on the body.[2]

PARSI WOMEN in addition tie a mathabanu (white piece of cloth) on head.[2]

INDIAN CHRISTIAN MALES usually wear pants and short coats.[2]

INDIAN CHRISTIANS FEMALES put on skirts and cover their head with chadar.[2]

DETERMINATION OF SEX

Why sex determination is important?

It is important in cases

i.   Relating to heirship,
ii.   Disposal of property, marriage, education, impotence, rape, divorce, etc.
iii. Identification in living or in dead (mainly in advance decomposition cases) bodies and
iv.   When sex appears ambiguous.

Identification of sex

Presumptive evidence about sex:

➢ Outward appearance of the person, the physical features
➢ General contours of the face, moustache and beard, evidence of shaving, length of head hair.
➢ Clothes, figure, habits and voice, etc.

Highly probable signs: external sexual structures like:

➢ Developed breast
➢ Appropriate muscular development
➢ The female distribution of body hair and subcutaneous fat
➢ The vagina in the female
➢ Absence of breast tissue, male distribution of hair, appropriate physical development and penis in the male are the most probable signs for the male sex.

Most certain signs: presence of ovaries (menstruation after puberty) in female and testes (seminal emission after puberty) in male is the most certain signs of sex. Before this period, in doubtful cases nuclear sexing and study of sex chromosomes will be help.

Determination of sex of an individual
A normal person has 46 chromosomes. The chromatin pattern in male is XY, and in female it is XX. The difficulty arises when there is ambiguity of the external genitalia and secondary sexual characters are unable to confirm the sex. The sex of a person can be determined from:
1. morphological examination
2. microscopic examination
3. hormone assay
4. gonadal biopsy
5. DNA profiling
6. Radiological investigation.

In the dead determination of sex is done by demonstration of the specific sex organs.
Highly probable and presumptive evidence is useful in,
➢ Highly decomposed bodies where the sex organs have disappeared,
➢ Grossly mutilated bodies,
➢ Portions of the body and
➢ Deliberate destruction of the sex organs.

Morphological examination
If the external genitalia are normal, then mere external examination is enough to determine the sex of an individual, and after puberty, the secondary sexual characters help to differentiate and confirm the sex. The various morphological differentiating physical features of human sex are mentioned in **table. 3.** Determination of sex from bones.

Table: 3 Differentiating points between male and female[1]

Feature	Male	Female
Built	Muscular, stronger	Less muscular, delicate
Height	More	Less
Scalp hairs	Shorter, coarser	Longer and finer
Eyebrow	Coarser and thicker	Fine and thin
Voice	Hoarse after puberty	Soft
Moustache and beard	Present	Absent or rudimentary
Hair on pinna	Present	Absent
Body hair grow over	Chest, abdomen and limb	May be seen over limbs

Pubic hairs	Thicker, coarser, extend upwards up to the navel rudimentary	Horizontal, covering only mons pubis, triangular in distribution
Breast	Rudimentary	Well development
Thyroid cartilage	Prominent, angle<90	Less prominent, angle>120
Shoulder and hip	Broader than hip	Hip broader than shoulder
Chest and abdomen	Chest dimension is more	Abdomen dimension is more
Gluteal region	Flat	Full and roundish
Forearm	Anteroposterior flat	Roundish
Thigh	Cylindrical	Conical
Wrist and ankle	Coarse and rough	Smooth and delicate
External genitalia	Scrotum, testis and penis	Labia, clitoris and vagina
Internal genitalia	Vas deferens, prostate, seminal vesicle, ejaculatory ducts	Ovaries, uterine tube and uerus

Microscopic examination

Sex chromatin test (nuclear sexing) for sex determination can be done by demonstrating Barr body and Davidson body, which are more with the female cells as a collection of chromatin as shown in fig. can be helpful. In the buccal smear, the percentage of nuclei having a chromatin body (Barrbody) ranges from zero to four in males and 20-80 in females.

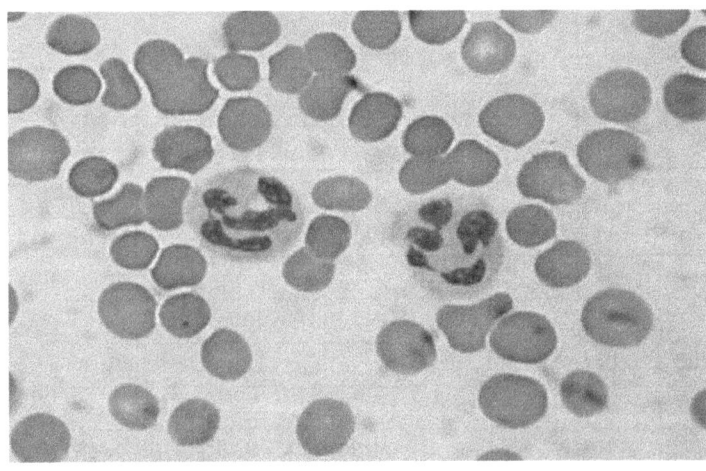

Barr body

The chromosomal study: the Y chromosome of the male cells can be visualized by using a fluorescent microscope and quinacrine hydrochloride stain in the cells of the hair sheaths, nerve cells and dental pulp.

Hormonal analysis
Hormonal imbalance will alter the secondary sexual characters and will confuse the determination of sex. Hormones are responsible for body contour, hairiness, fat distribution and genital morphology.

Gonadal biopsy
The gonadal biopsy provides essential information for the identification, besides classification and early detection of neoplasias in patients with disorders of sex development. A biopsy from the gonads, if indicates testis in male and ovary in female, is the definite identity of the sex of the person.

DNA profiling
DNA profiling can determine the sex of a person from blood stains or even from fragmentary remains.Troubles in sex determination

Troubles in sex determination
- Concealed sex
- Decomposed or mutilatedbodies
- Skeleton
- Intersex state.[1, 2, 3]

Concealed sex
Concealed or hidden sex is the lack of distinctive signaling that an individual may show to hide his or her sex for some criminal motives or some other objects, etc. criminal may conceal their sex to avoid detection by changing dress or other methods. This can be detected by proper physical examination.

Sex from decomposed or mutilated bodies
When the body is found in the advanced putrefaction state, sex can be determined by the presence of either uterus or prostate, which resist putrefaction for a long time.

Sex from skeleton
It is not possible to determine from skeleton the full amount of certainty till puberty, since the sexual characteristics of the bone begin to manifest only after attainment of puberty. Only exception is the pelvis where the greater sciatic notch can be utilized for sex determination in children.

Intersex state[1, 2, 3]
Types of intersex: it is mixing of characters of both sexes in one individual in varying degrees, including physical form, reproductive organs and sexual behavior as a result of some defect in the embryonic development. It can be categorized into four groups
- Gonadal agencies
- Gonadal dysgenesis
- True hermaphroditism

➢ Pseudohermaphroditism[1,2,3]

Klinefelter syndrome

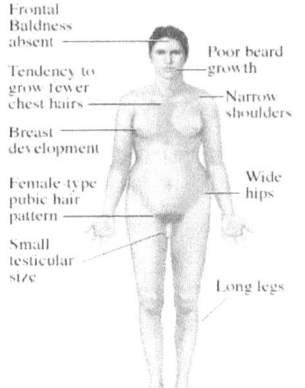

Frontal
Baldness
absent

Poor beard
growth

Tendency to
grow fewer
chest hairs

Narrow
shoulders

Breast
development

Female-type
pubic hair
pattern

Wide
hips

Small
testicular
size

Long legs

- **Lower IQ than sibs**

- **Tall stature**

- **Poor muscle tone**

- **Reduced secondary sexual characteristics**

- **Gynaecomastia (male breasts)**

- **Small testes/infertility**

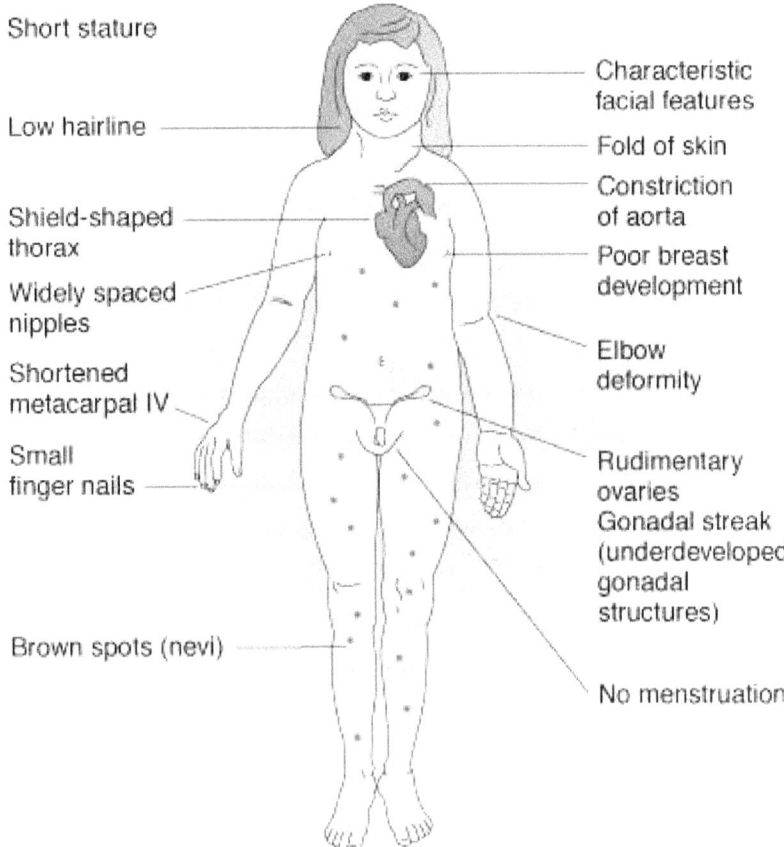

Short stature

Low hairline

Shield-shaped thorax

Widely spaced nipples

Shortened metacarpal IV

Small finger nails

Brown spots (nevi)

Characteristic facial features

Fold of skin

Constriction of aorta

Poor breast development

Elbow deformity

Rudimentary ovaries
Gonadal streak (underdeveloped gonadal structures)

No menstruation

Turner's syndrome

Gonadal agencies[1,2]

In this condition, testes or the ovaries have never developed and nuclear sexing is negative.

Gonadal dysgenesis[1,2]

Here, the external sexual structures are present but they fail to develop at puberty and have no gonads. The examples are: Klinefelter's syndrome and Turner's syndrome.

Klinefelter's syndrome

In this condition, anatomical structure is male, but the nuclear sexing is female. The study reveals the presence of two X chromosomes in combination with one Y chromosomes, the sex chromosome pattern is XXY (47 chromosomes) the incidence of this syndrome is 1:500, and it increases with advancing maternal age. It is diagnosed when there is delayed onset of puberty, behavioral disorders and mental retardation. Hair on the chest and chin are reduced with absence of axillary and pubic hair. Gynecomastia, azoospermia, low levels of testosterone, sterility, increased urinary gonadotropin and increased height are commonly seen. Histologically, there is atrophy of the testicles with hyalinization of seminiferous tubules.

Turner's syndrome

In this condition, the anatomical structure is female, but nuclear sexing is male. The cytogenetic study shows monosomy X, the sex chromosome pattern is XO. It can be diagnosed at birth by the presence of edema of hand and feet, loose skin folds at the nape of the neck, low birth weight and short stature.

It is characterizes by primary amenorrhea, sterility, lack of development of primary and secondary sexual characteristics, infantile streak ovaries, increased urinary gonadotropin excretion, short fourth metatarsal, webbed neck, shield-chest, wide straight nipples, high arched plate, low set ears, slow growth, learning problems. It is also associated with other congenital malformation like color blindness, spina bifida, coarctation of the aorta, septal Defects, renal defects like horseshoe kidney, endocrinological defects like Cushing'ssyndrome and high incidence of diabetes mellitus.

True hermaphroditism

It has both gonadal organs, i.e. +ve test. It is a very rare condition. The person will be having internal and external gonads of both sexes and be able to function as either a male or a female, depending on how he or she has been brought up initially.

The gonads may be abdominal, inguinal, labioscrotal in position. The phallus may be penile or clitoral; labia may be bifid as in female or fused resembling the scrotum of the male. Neither gonad is functional; histology reveals both testicular and ovarian tissues.[1]

Pseudohermaphroditism

Sex determined from the gonads, nuclear sex gives true sex. In this condition, the presence of gonadal tissue of only one sex is seen internally, while the external appearance is of the opposite sex. It is of two types male and female:

> Male pseudohermaphroditism
> Female pseudohermaphroditism[1, 2, 3]

Male pseudohermaphroditism

Nuclear sexing is XY, but sex organs and sexual characteristics deviate towards female form because of testicular feminization. There is the inability to convert testosterone into active form dihydro-testosterone. Organs and sexual characteristics towards male are seen due to adrenal hyperplasia.

Female pseudohermaphroditism

Female pseudo hermaphrodites are chromosomally and gonadally female, but have male or ambiguous external genitalia. There is a variable degree of clitoral hypertrophy and labial fusion. The ovaries are sometimes cystic. Secondary sexual characteristics may also show virilization or poor feminization. Female pseudohermaphroditism is caused by excess of androgen, e.g. testosterone of extra gonadal origin. It is an uncommon condition and found with ratio of <1:10,000. [1]

DETERMINATION OF AGE[1]

Age estimation is an important activity that is frequently required to be carried out by a medico legal expert. An individual is often referred to a medical man by the court or investigating authority in criminal as well as in civil cases to give the option regarding his or her age. Forensic age estimation in living subjects has gained increasing significance in recent years. Determination of age is required in the fetus, children and adult and even in dead bodies including skeletal remains.

The following data are utilized for determination of age[1]:

I.   Psychological data
II.   Physical data
III. Dental data
IV.   Radiological data
V.   Other sensile changes

First 7to 10 days after conception, i.e.Until the implantation occurs the term developing ovum is fused. It is called an 'embryo' from one week to the end of the second month, and later it is called a fetus.it becomes an infant when it is completely born. Table:4

Table: 4 different periods of infants[1]

Prenatal period:ovum or zygote form from zero day to 14 days; embryo form from14 days to 8 weeks, fetus form from 9 weeks to birth

> **Perinatal period:**It is the time period pertaining to the period immediately before and after birth. The perinatal period is an interval extending approximately from the 28th week of gestation to the 28th day after birth

> **Postnatal period:**postnatal a Latin word means after birth (from post, meaning after and natalis, means birth) is the period beginning immediately after the birth of a child and extending for about 6 weeks. The term postpartum period. Refers to the mother, whereas postnatal refers to the infant

Age of the fetus [1]
Age of a fetus can be assessed as follows:
- Crown –heel length
- Crown-rump length
- Weight
- Physical features
- Appearance of epiphyseal center

Length and weight[1]
The male infants weigh about 100g more than the female. The circumference ofthe head is 33-36 cm. at full term, the head of a child is nearly one-fourth of the whole length of the body. The surface of the brain shows convolutions, and the gray matter begins to form.

The scalp hair is dark, 3 or 5 cm long, the face is not wrinkled. Lanugo is absent except on the shoulders. The skin us pale and covered with vernix caseosa.

The nails project beyond the end of fingers, but reach only the tip of the toes. The cartilages are formed in the nose and ears. The testes arepresent in the scrotum;vulvaisclosed labia minora are covered by fully developed labia majora. The rectum contains dark brownish, green or black meconium.

The placenta is 22cm in diameter, one and half cm thick at the center, and weight about 500g.the umbilicus is situated midway between the pubis and xiphoid cartilage. The umbilical cord is 50-55 cm long and one cm thick .the center of ossification is found in the lower end of the femur and sometimes in the cuboids and in the upper end of the tibia. Six fontanelles are usually present in the neonatal skull.

Rule of haase[1]
This is rough method of calculating the age of the fetus .the length of the fetus is measured from the crown to the heel in cm. during the first 5 months ofpregnancy, the square root of the length gives the approximate age of the fetus in the months, e.g., a fetus of 16 cm is of 4 months duration .until the fetus reaches the length of 25 cm, the square root of the crown-heel length is taken to arrive at the age.

When the length of the fetus is more than 25 cm,it is divided by five .hence, for the last months, the length in cm divided by five give the age in months, e .g fetus of 35 cm in 7 months.

Physical features[1]

End of first month

length 1 cm ; weight 2.5 g ,the eyes are seen as two dark spots and the moth as a cleft nucleated red cells begin to form in the placenta.

End of second month

Length 1cm; weight 10 g. the hands and feet are webbed, the placenta begins to form.   The anus is seen as   dark spot first ossification center in a fetus appears in clavicle (4 to 5 weeks), followed by maxilla (6 weeks).

End of third month

Length 9 cm; weight   30-35g. Theeyes are closed, the pupillary membrane appears. Nails appear in membranous form and the neck is formed.

End of fourth month

Length 16cm; weight 120-130g. At this stage sex can be recognized. Lanugo hair is en on the body. Convolutions begin to develop in the brain. Meconium is found in the duodenum

End of fifth month

Length 25 cm; weight 400g nails are distinct and soft and up to a proximityof fingers Light hair appears on the head .skin is covered with vernix caseosa. Meconioum is seen at the beginning of the large intestine. Center for manubrium, 1st segment of sternum are seen .

End of sixth month

Length 30 cm; weight 700g eyebrows , eyelashes appear and adherent . Skin is red and wrinkled and subcutaneous fat begins to be deposited .the testes are seen close to the kidneys .sylvian fissure of the brain is formed . Meconium is in transverse colon .

End of seventh month

Length 35cm; crown –rump length 23 cm ; foot length 8 cm; weight 900-1200g. Nails are up to tips of fingers. Eyelids open and pupillary membrane disappears. Skin is dusky red , thick and fibrous. Meconium is found in the entire large intestine .testes is found at the external inguinal ring . Gallbladder contains bile and cecum is seen in the right iliac fossa. Ossification center for talus appears.

End of eighth month

Length 40cm; weight 1.5 kg Nails reach the tips of fingers. Scalp hair is thicker. Skin is not wrinkled. Left testis is present in the scrotum. Placenta weighs 500g.

End of ninth month

Length 45cm; weight 2.5-3 kg. Scalp hair is dark and 4 cm long. Meconium is seen at the end of large intestine. Scrotum is wrinkled and contains both testis. Placenta weighs 500g. Ossification centers are usually present in the lower and of femur.

End of tenth month (full term child)

Length 50-53 cm; crown-rump length 30-33cm; weight 2.5-5 kg; the length is much less variable than the weight. Different age related changes in the fetus are briefed in table: 5

Table:5 Age- related changes in the fetus[1]

Month (IUL)	Three months	Four months	Five months	Six months	Seven months	Eight months	Nine months
Length (cm)	9	16	25	30	35	40	45
Weight	30-35g	120-130g	400g	700g	900-1200g	1.5kg	2-2.5kg
Nails	Present in membranous form	-	Up to proximity of tip of finger	-	Up to tip of finger	-	Beyond the tip of the finger
Hairs	-	Lanugos appears	Scalp hairs appears	-	Scalp hair 1cm long	Scalp hair 1.5cm	Scalp hair 2cm
Sex	-	Distinguishable	-	Well distinguished	-	-	-
Eyelids	-	-	-	Adherent and eye lashes present	Non adherent and eye lashes present	Well formed	-
Brain	-	-	-	-		-	-
Intestine	-	Meconium in upper part of small intestine	Meconium up to ascending colon	Meconium in transverse colon	Meconium in descending pelvic colon	-	Meconium in rectum
Scrotum	-	-	-	Empty	-	Corrugated	Occupied testis

Testes	-	-	-	On psoas muscle	Near the internal inguinal ring	In canal(L >R)	Inside scrotum
Centers of ossification	-	-	Manubrium 1st segment of sternum	-	Talus and 2nd and 3rd segments of sternum	-	Lower end of femur and cuboid

Appearances of ossification center [1]

1. **Sternum:** it is placed flat on a wooden board and cut with the cartilages knife in its long axis in midline, which exposes the ossifications centers
2. **Lower end of the femur and upper end of the tibia:** The legs flexed against the thigh and a transverse or vertical incision is made into the knee joint. The patella is removed. The end of the femur is pushed forward through the wound ,end a number of parallel cross-sections are made through the epiphysis starting from its articular surface and continuing until the largest part of ossification center is reach The center is seen as a brownish red nucleus surrounded by bluish white Cartilage above it until the diaphyseal center is reached.The center appears in about the 36th week. Its diameter is about 4-5 mm And 37-38 weeks and 6-8mm at full term, the upper end of tibia is similarly Examined.
3. **Bones of the foot:** the foot grasped in the left hand behind the heel,The toes pointing towards dissector. An incision is made between the interspaces of third and fourth toes with a long knife , backwards through the sole of the foot and heel. If center in calcaneum andtalus are not exposed,Thin slices of cartilages of these bones should be cut until presence or absence has been shown. Center in the calcaneum appears at the end of the seventh month of intrauterine life. A center may be present in cuboid at birth, or it may appear shortly afterwards.

Age from birth till 25 years

Physical examination for Age estimation

➢ An approximate age of a person can be estimated from height and weight.

➢ Development of secondary sexual characteristics like axillary and pubic hair,

➢ Growth of bread and moustache, development of secondary sexual organs

➢ And menstrual history, etc. , can be of added help. Feature of graying hair,

> Balding, decrease in stature, changes in the skin, arcus senilis,   corneal
> Opacity ,cataract, etc. Give an idea of advancing age.

Secondary sexual characters: these develop at the time of puberty due to the influence of hormones and are useful for the determination of age at that period. The voice becomes deep due to elongation of the vocal cords. This change is more prominently seen in boys than in girls. Fine hair begins to appear on the penis. The development of pubic hair and genital organs can be assessed by **tanner staging,** which divides it into five stages as follows:

In boys

Stage 1: no pubic hairs and penis and testicles are in the same proportion as in childhood.

Stage 2: spare growth of long, slightly darkened, pubic hair at the base of the penis is seen. The   testicles begin to get larger, and the scrotum begins to get reddened and altered texture, the penis may grow slightly .

Stage 3: pubic hair gets darker, coarser and curlier. It begins to spread over pubic bone the testicles continue to enlarge and the scrotum texture becomes more like that of an adult. The penis gets longer.

Stage 4: pubic hair grows to cover the base of penis and begins to grow on the upper part of scrotum. The hair gets darker , coarser and curlier. The scrotal skin gets darker as the testicles continue to grow. The penis continues to grow longer and gets wider. The glans or head, of the penis becomes much more prominent.

Stage 5: pubic has hair gets spread to inside of the thighs. The scrotum,testicles and penis grow to their final adult size and shape.Development of axillary hair, beard and moustache and body hair takes place subsequently.

In girls

Stage 1: No pubic hair

Stage 2: There is sparse growth of long, slightly darkened, downy hair mostly long the labia. This hair is usually straight or slightly curled.

Stage 3: Hair becomesdarker, coarser and curlier. It now grows sparsely over the mons veneris area.

Stage 4: Hair growths are seen more densely. It becomes as coarse and curly as in the adult, but does not extend onto the inner thighs.

Stage 5: Classic, coarse and curly pubic hair that extend up to inner thighs.

Tanner staging of breast   development is as follows[1]:

Stage1: Small elevated nipple with no significant underlying tissue.

Stage 2: Elevation of breast and nipple as small mound; the areola begins to enlarge.

Stage 3: Further enlargementand elevationof the breast and areola (with no separation of their contours) takes place. The areola begins to darken in color.

Stage 4: Projection of the areola and nipple to form secondary mound.

Stage 5: Mature adultbreast, there is a projection of nipple only,Development of axillary hair and body hair takes place subsequently.

Dental examination for age estimation[1]

In dental age estimation, tooth eruption is a parameter of developmental morphology that can be analyzed by either clinical examination or by evaluation of dental x ray.

The three stages of human dentition, viz. deciduous or temporary, mixed and permanent follow a periodic sequence that can be utilized for estimation of age of different accuracy.

Radiological examination for age estimation[1]

This procedure is used to know:
- appearance and fusion of ossification centers
- study of diaphyseal length
- calcification of root of teeth

Appearance and fusion of ossification centers[1]

Radiological data are accepted to be the most reliable. The appearance and union ossification centers follow a definite time sequence, which can be utilized for the age estimation. However, following common features should be remembered while opining the age from radiological finding if bone:

Common features
- Radiological data can be easily be determined by studying appearances of ossification centers and their fusion with the adjacent centers by radiological examination of the bones.
- The bones of the whole skeleton develop from the performed hyaline cartilage by the process of **" osteogenesis ".**
- Large numbers of ossification centers appear in the performed cartilage at different periods of life. At 11-12th week of intrauterine life, there 806 ossification centers, at birth, they are about 450 and an adult skeleton contains only 206 bones.
- Usually in epiphyses, ossification starts centrally and then spreads to the periphery.
- At the start with, the centers are small , rounded, size of a pinhead, as it grows it takes the shape of the bone.
- Small bones like , carpal, tarsal bones grow from single center , where as long bones grow from multiple centers.
- Increase in length of long bones occurs in the layered cartilage persisting in between the diaphysis and epiphysis, until it attains the adult shape and size.
- Shaft or diaphysis of most of the long bones develops from one center, while the ends or the epiphysis are developed from separate centers. These epiphyseal centers are secondary centers.
- Both the terminal ends of the long bones of the limbs develop from separate ossification centers, while the ends of the bones like clavicle, rib and metacarpal, metatarsal develop from one epiphysis at one end only .
- Epiphyseal union occurs 1 to2 years earlier in females than males.
- Epiphyseal union is earlier in tropical countries than in temperate zones.

The time of bony epiphyseal union is not same throughout India . it differs even up to 2-3 years from south to north ,east to west. Shown in table 6.

In young children , radiological examination of hand and foot alone can give an accurate estimation of age, but in adult two or three joints ,viz. wrist, elbow , shoulder, hip, knee and ankle joint and skull (anteroposteriorand lateral view) are to be radiographed , depending upon the person's age. Chest with sternoclavicular joints in anteroposterior and chest with sternum and vertebrae is to be x-rayed in a lateral view position for the purpose of age estimation.

Table .6 Centers of ossification as observed by galstaun in Indian subjects[1]

Bone/joint (A- Appear, F-fusion)	Female	Male
Clavicle (sternal end)	A 14-16 years F 20 years	A 15-19 years F 22 years
Base of coracoid of scapula	A 25 months F 25 years	A 25 months F 25 years
Coracoid of scapula	A 10-11 years F 16 years	A 10-11 years F 16years
Angle of coracoid of scapula	A 8-10 years F16 years	A 10-14 years F 17-18 years
Acromion of scapula	A 12- 14 years F 13-16 years	A 14-17 F 14-19 years
Head of humerus	A 1st year F 14- 16	A 1st year F 14- 18 years
Greater tubercle of humerus (fusion to head)	A 7 month- 4 years F 2-4	A 7 month- 4 years F 2-4 years
Greater tubercle of humerus (fusion to lesser tubercle)	A 7 months- F 5-7 years	A 7 month F 5-7 years
Trochlea fusion to capitulum	A10 year F 9-13 years	A 11 years F 11-15 years
Lateral epicondyle fusion to capitulum	A 10 years F 10- 12 years	A 11 years F 11- 16 years
Medial epicondyle fusion to shaft distal humeral epiphysis	A5 years F14 years	A 7 years F 16 years
Radius, head	A6 years F14 years	A 8 years F 16 years
Radius, distal end	A 1 years F 16.5 years	A 1 years F16 -17 years
Ulna, olecranon	A 9-12 years F 15 years	A 11-13 years F17 years
Ulna, distal end	A 8-10 years F 17 years	A 10- 11 years F 18 years
Hip bone, iliac crest	A 14 years F 17- 19 years	A 17 years F 19- 20 years

Hip bone, ischium and pubis	A F 8.5 years	A F 8.5 years
Acetabulum: disappearance of triradiate cartilage	14 years	15 16 years
Ischial tuberosity of hip bone	A 14- 16 years F 20 years	A 16-18 years F 20 years
Head of femur	A 1st years F 14- 15 years	A 1st year F 16-17 years
Greater trochanter of femur	A 3 years F 14 years	A 3 years F 17 years
Lesser trochanter of femur	A 1st year F 15- 17 years	A 1st years F 15- 17 years
Distal end of femur	A before birth F 14- 17 years	A before birth F 14- 17 years
Proximal end of tibia	A shortly before or after birth F 14-15 years	A shortly before or after birth F 15-17 years
Distal end of tibia	A F 14.1-14.4 years	A F 16 years
Proximal end of fibula	A F 14- 16 years	A F 11-16 years
Distal end of fibula	A F 13- 15 years	A F 14- 16 years
Patella	A 4 years	A 3-4 years
Carpal bone, Capitate	A ½ years	A 1/2years
Hamate	A 8-14 month	A 8-14 months
Triquetral	A 2-3 years	A 3- 4 years
Lunate	A 5 years	A 5 years
Trapezium	A 5-6 years	A 7 years
Trapezoid	A 5-6 years	A 4-7 years
Scaphoid	A 6 years	A 7-11 years
Pisiform	A 9-12 years	A 12- 17 years
First metacarpal bone	A 3 years F 14-15 years	A 4 years F 16- 18 years

2nd, 3rd, 4th and 5th metacarpal bones	A 2-3 years F 14- 15 year	A 3-4 years F 16-18 years
phalanges of hand, proximal row	A 5 years F 14-15 years	A 2-4 years F 17-18 years
Phalanges of hand, middle row	A 2-3 years F 14- 16 years	A 3 years F 16- 18 years
Phalanges of hand, terminal row	A 3 years F 15 years	A 3-5 years F 17 18 years
Tarsal bone, calcaneum and talus	A at birth	A at birth
Cuboid	Aat birth	A at birth
Internal cuneiform	A 1-3 years	A 1-4 years
Middle cuneiform	A 1-3 years	A 2-4 years
External cuneiform	A 1-3 years	A 1-4 years
Navicular	A 1-3 years	A 1-4 years
1st metatarsal	A 3 years F 14- 15 years	A 4-5 years F 16-18 years
2nd, 3rd, 4th and 5th metatarsal	A 3 years F 14- 15 years	A 4-5 years F 16-18 yeas
Tarsal phalanges, proximal row	A 1-3 years F 14-15 years	A 3-4 years F 16-18 years
middle row	A 3-4 years F 14-15 years	A 3-4 years F 16-18 years
Terminal row	A 4-6 years F 13-14 years	A 4-6 years F 15-17 years

As a rule the ageing of bones is more accurate with the appearance of ossification centers than the unions of same. In the long bones of upper limbs, the union is earlier at the elbow joint and later at the wrist joint. Head of the humerus is the last long bone epiphysis to unite in the upper limb. In the lower limb, union occurs earlier at the tip and ankle joints and later at the knee joint.

The **epiphyseal plate** is a hyaline cartilage plate in the metaphysis at each end of a long bone. The plate is found in children and adolescents; in adults , who have stopped growing, the plate is replaced by an **epiphyseal line** . The epiphyseal lines on the long bones of a young individual appear as circular grooves around the ends of the bones , and on x-rays, it appears as irregular lines resembling a fracture. When bones are dried , the epiphysis may be separated in a young child from the shaft, which should not be mistaken for fractures. Skeletal age is based on appearance and union of epiphyseal centers, which should be expressed as plus or minus some years.

The process of fusion of epiphyseal with diaphysis is called **"union".** Union may beinterpreted as (a) not united (b) uniting, all on the basis of stage of union. The radiological bony union is 2-3 years earlier than anatomical bony union. This is due to the fact ,that towards the end of the growth period , the epiphyseal plate of the hyaline cartilage becomes thin and irregular in outlines called epiphyseal line , which may not be detected on X – ray . In x-ray plate, persistent scar is neither the evidence of incomplete union not the recent union.[1]

Disturbance in skeletal growth and maturation[1]

The relationship of the endocrine glands to skeletal growth and maturation is very important. Roentgen examination of the growing skeleton may give valuable information concerning thyroid, pituitary and gonadal disturbances. They all cause generalized skeletal age abnormality. Delay in appearance or fusion or retardation of epiphyseal centers may result from deficient secretion of one or more of these glands. Hypersecretion may accelerate this process.

Graham CB[4]in his study indicates a number of glandular disturbances and their effect on skeletal maturation. Focal increases in maturation may occur following infection, burns, frostbites, radiation therapy or trauma, particularly epiphyseal separations. These   all impair the growth potential   either by destroying the resting cells or by disrupting the blood supply and growth may cease. Premature closure of the epiphysis may occur as the result of bone infracts, particularly in sickle cell disease, some important X-ray plates are shown in fig. from A to L commonly used for the purpose of age estimation .

Apart from X-rays, computed tomography of head for suture closure ectocranially can also be done. The most reliable estimation of age is from ectocranial union of suture and the order of accuracy is: sagittal, lambdoid and then coronal.

Agesfrom **skeletal** changes and **histological** age estimation from bone are discussed in the forensic osteology.

Medicolegal importance of age[1]

> ➤ **Above seven months of intrauterine**: Viability is attained**.** Under section 302of IPC, charge of infanticide is leveled.
> ➤ **Five years of age:** (1) according to section 6 (a) of " the Hindu minority and guardianship act, 1956", a minor who has not completed the age of 5 years shall ordinarily be in the custody of the mother ; (2) half fare in railway ; (3) child is held responsible for any wreckage caused to train (as per railway act).
> ➤ **Criminal responsibility:** Any act done by a child under 7 years of age is not an offence (section 82 IPC). A child between 7 and 12 years is presumed to be capable of committing an offence, if he has attained sufficient maturity of understanding to judge the nature and consequences of his conduct on that occasion (section 83 IPC). This maturity is presumed in a child unless otherwise proved by defense. A child under 12 years of age cannot give valid consent to suffer any harm, which may occur from an act done in good faith and for its benefit (section 89 IPC). A person above 18 years can give valid consent to

suffer any harm, which may result from an act not known to cause death or grievous hurt (section 87 IPC).

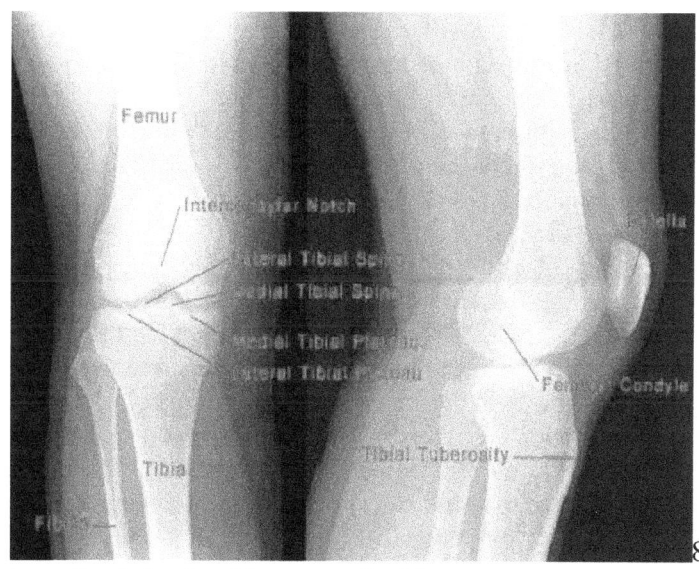

Knee joint union of epiphysis of lower end of femur and upper end of tibia and fibula, age below 17

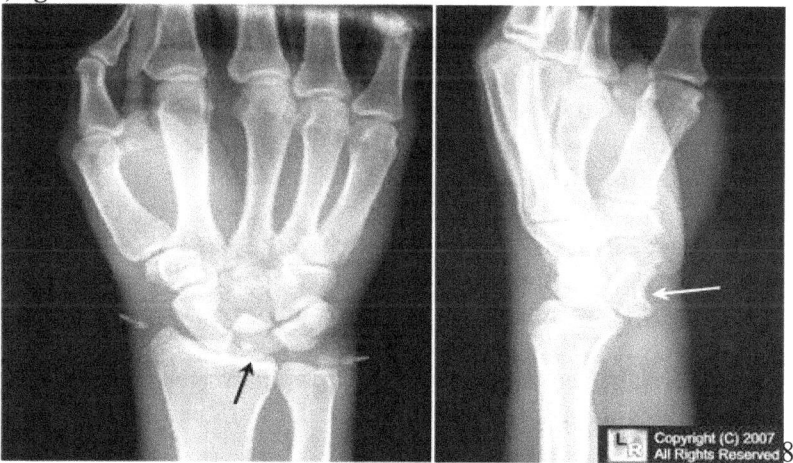

Wrist and hand showing lower epiphysis of first metcarpal is not united with shaft.age12-15

Medicolegal Importance of Age

> **Judicial punishment:** According to **the juvenile justice**(care and protection of children) act 2000,' juvenile or boy 'means a person who has not completed 18 years of age. the juvenile justice board may advise or admonish the juvenile or order to participate in group counseling or perform community service or to be released on probation of conduct or to pay a fine or to make an order directing the juvenile to be sent to a

53

special home for the period until he becomes major. No juvenile found guilty by law shall be sentenced to death or life imprisonment or committed to prison.[1, 2, 3]

> **Rape :**sexual intercourse by a man with a girl under 15 years , even if she is his own wife (by local amendment this age has been reduced to 13 years for the state of Manipur), or with any other girl under 16 years even with her consent is rape (section 375 IPC).[1,3] However, anti-rape bill has been passed in lok sabha on **19th march, 2013,** which provides that theage of consent for sex would be 18 years.

> **Employment:**A child below 14 years of age cannot be employed to work in a factory or mine or in many other risky employments. A child between 14 and 15 years of age can be engaged in non –hazardous factory-jobs for a limited period during the day hours,. A person who has completed 15 years is allowed to work in a factory as an adult if a fitness certificate is issued to him by a certifying surgeon.

> **Kidnapping:** In criminal law**, kidnapping**is the taking away or transportation of a person against the person's will, usually to hold the person in false imprisonment (a confinement without legal authority). It is an offence to kidnap a (1) child with the intension of taking dishonesty any movable property, if the age is under 10 years (section 369 IPC); (2) minor from lawful guardianship if the age of a boy is under 16 years and that of a girl under 18 years (section 366 IPC); (3) girl for prostitution, if her age is below 18 years (section 366-a, IPC) and (4) girl to import into India from a foreign country for purposes of eliciting intercourse, if her age is less than 21 years (section 366-b).[1,2,3]

> **Attainment of majority:** as per section 3of the Indian majority act, 1875, a person attains majority on the completion of 18th years, but if a person is under a guardianship of the court of wards (under a guardian appointed by the court), he attains majority on the completion of 21 years.

> **Evidence:**competency **for** giving evidence depends upon age. Section 118 of IEA states that a person of any age can give evidence if the court is satisfied that the child is truthful.

> **Marriage contract:**As per child marriage restraint act 1978, the minimum age of marriage for females is 18 years and that for males is 21 years.

> **Criminal abortion:**one cannot**charge** a woman**for** procuring criminal abortion for a woman who has passed childbearing age.[1, 2, 3, 5, 6]

> **Infanticide:**if the infant is under the age of 7 months of intrauterine life, then the charge of infanticide cannot be supported.[1,2,3,5]

> **Identification:**An approximate age is important in any identification data.

> **Impotence and sterility:**a boy is sterile before puberty, though notimpotent. Women become sterile after menopause.

> **Importance of 25 years of age:**

- According to article 84(b) of the constitution of India, minimum age for contesting for the membership of parliament is 25 years.
- According to article 173(b) of the constitution , minimum age for contesting for the membership of any state legislative assembly is 25 years.
- This is the maximum age for any entry into some government services.
- According to Punjab excise act 1914, a person below this age cannot buy and consume liquor.

➢ **Importance of 30 years of age:**
- According to article 84(b) of the constitution of India, this is the minimum age for election to the state legislative council.
- According to article 173(b) this is the minimum age for election to the state legislative council.

➢ **Importance of 35 years of age:**
- According to article 58(1(B) of the constitution of India, this is the minimum age for appointment as the president of India.
- According to article 66(3(B), this the minimum age for appointment as the vice –president of India.
- According to article 157, this is the minimum age for appointment as the governor of any state.
- According to section 43(i) of the parental diagnostic techniques (regulation and prevention of misuse) ac 1994. No parental diagnostic technique shall be used or conducted unless the age of the woman is above 35 years.

➢ **Importance of 60 years of age:** this is the age of retirement from government service.

➢ **Importance of 65 years of age:** according to section 10 (2) of the consumer protection act 1986, every member of the district forum shall hold office for a term of 5 years or up to the age of 65 years , whichever is earlier, and shall not eligible for reappointment . district forum is a kind of civil court, which delivers judgments, in cases of consumer grievances. Similarly, the state commission and the national commission are also akin to civil courts, which are higher in rank to district forum.

➢ **Importance of 67 years of age:**according to section 16 (3) of the consumer protection act 1986, every member of the state commission shall be below 67 years of age.

➢ **Importance of 70 years:**according to section 20 (3) of the consumer protection act 1986, every member of the national commission shall be below 70 years of age. This is the age prescribed by some state governments, which qualifies a person to get pension from "old age pension scheme."

STATURE

Stature means body height of a person. It shows a **diurnal variation** by half to two cm.it is less in the afternoon and evening due to the reduced elasticity of the intervertebral discs and the longitudinal vertebral muscles. Both malnutrition and advancing years reduce stature. After the age of 30, the natural processes of senile degeneration cause gradual decrease in stature by about 0.6 mm per year on an average. The stature is greater by 1-3 cm on lying. Due to complete loss of muscle tone, relaxation of large joints and loss of tensioning effect of Para-spinal muscles on intervertebral discs, the body shows lengthening after death by about two cm.

Stature of dismembered body

In case of **dismembered body,** the approximate **stature is determined** as follows:

1. The length from the tip of the middle finger to the tip of the opposite middle finger, when arms are fully extended, approximately equals the height.
2. Twice the length of one arm, with 30 cm added for two clavicles and four cm for the sternum, is equal to the height.
3. The length from the vertex to the symphysis is roughly half of stature.
4. The length from the sternal notch to symphysis pubis multiplied by 3.3 gives the stature.
5. The length of forearm measured from tip of olecranon process to tip of the middle finger is equal to 5/19 of the stature.
6. The height of head measured by the vertical distance from the top of the head to the tip of the chin is about one-seventh of the total height.
7. The length of vertebral column is 35/100 of the height.
8. To the length of entire skeleton add two –and-half to four cm for the thickness of the soft parts.
9. Maximum foot length divided by 0.15 gives stature.[1]

ANTHROPOMETRY (BERTILLON SYSTEM)

The science of measuring the body parts constitutes Bertillon system or anthropometry.

Principle

After the age of 21 years, the skeleton stops growing. Hence the dimensions of the skeleton remain unchanged and that the ratio in size of different parts to one another varies considerably in different individuals. As such, this can be applied only to adults. This system includes recordings of:

➤ **Descriptive data:** such as color of hair, eyes, complexion, and shape of nose.
➤ **Body marks:** such as moles, scars, tattoo marks.
➤ **Body measurements:** such as height, anteroposterior diameter of head and trunk, the span of outstretched arms, the length of left middle finger, left little finger, left forearm, left foot, length and breadth of right ear and color of left iris. The photographs of a front view of the head, a profile view of the right side of head are also taken. Though photographs are very useful means of identification, they are not free from errors. This system has now been replaced by dactylography.

FINGERPRINT SYSTEM

This is also known as dactylography or dermatoglyphics or Galton system.

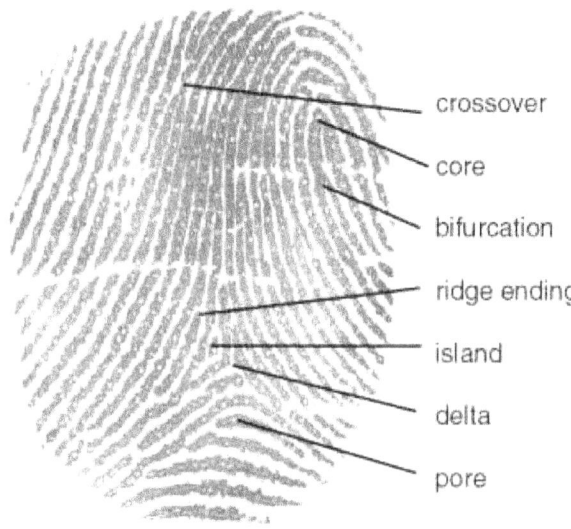

crossover
core
bifurcation
ridge ending
island
delta
pore

Definition

Fingerprints are impressions of patterns formed by the papillary or epidermal ridge of the finger tips. At birth, a fine pattern of ridges Is seen on the skin of the bulbs of the fingers and thumbs, parts of the palms and the soles of the feet.[1]

Are impressions of the balls of the fingers and thumbs either detected at a scene of crime or recorded by moistening the skin with printer's ink and pressing or rolling on prepared paper so that a permanent record results.[4]

Principal of use

The skin of the fingerprints is covered with ridges on which the sweat pores open in certain characters that are specific for each person. The pattern is absolutely individual, as it develops at the 16th weeks of intrauterine life and remains constant for life no two person's fingerprints are exactly alike, not even those of identical twins.

Fingerprints are present in both epidermis and dermis, and so, they are not destructed by the peeling of the superficial epithelium that may occur in early submersion under water or putrefaction. Fingerprints are transiently lost in exposure to ionizing radiation, but permanently lost in surgical removal, chemical destruction, chronic skin diseases, e.g. leprosy and by LASER leaving no scar for identification.[1]

Histological background

I.   Clay tablets from ancient Babylonia indicate the first civilizations to have attempted to identify criminals by their fingerprints. As early as 200 BC, the Chinese used fingerprints as a personal signature. The use of fingerprint in record in official documents of china dates back to 3000 BC.

II. It is stated that the first scientific study on fingerprint was done by **professor melphige in 1680.**

III. **Sir William Herschel,** working in the Hooghly district of Bengal, used palm prints
Of Indian people for identifying them legally. Herschel, a British officer in India in the 1850s, is credited with the first systematic use of fingerprints for identification. Fingerprints Bureau was first established in Kolkata.

- The first system that allowed fingerprints to be matched against each other in an efficient manner was devised by Sir Francis Galton, an English scientist, in 1892. He also published his work in the form of a book 'fingerprint'.
- His system was modified and implemented in criminal investigations by **Sir Edward Henry,** a commissioner of Scotland Yard in London, in 1901. The Henry system is used in most countries today. Some South American countries, however, use a system devised by Juan Vucetich, an Argentine.Fingerprintswere first used in US in 1903 in New York state prisons. The federal bureau of investigation (FBI) has maintained its central file since 1924. FBI holds the largest collection of fingerprints.[1]

Classification

Sir Galtonclassified fingerprint into four major or primary types based types based on the arrangement of papillary ridges:

- **Arches:** comprising 6-7% of all prints. The ridges go from one side of the finger to the other.
- **Loops:**about 67%. The ridges make a background turn in their course from one side of the finger to the other. This turn may be radial (3%) or ulnar (65%).
- **Composite:** A combination of one or more of the previous types. It comprises 1-2% of all prints. It is further subdivided into (a) central pocket loops, (B) lateral pocket loops, (c) twinned loops, (D) accidentals.
- **Whorls:** the ridges make one or more than complete turn. It comprises 25% of all prints. It is further categorized into (A) concentric (B) spiral,(c) double spiral,(d) almond –shaped.[1,2,3,4]

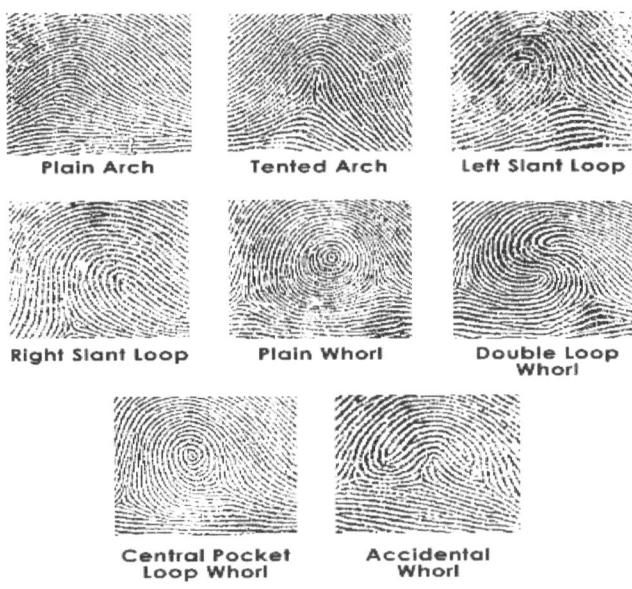

Plain Arch   Tented Arch   Left Slant Loop

Right Slant Loop   Plain Whorl   Double Loop Whorl

Central Pocket Loop Whorl   Accidental Whorl

Loops usually begin on side of the finger and can be further of radial or ulnar subtypes. In a whorl, the ridges form a series of circles or spirals around the core. Whorl, can be concentric, spiral, double spiral or almond-shaped. Arches are wave like pattern from one side to the other side and may have subtypes like plain, tented and exceptional.in a composite variety may include the central pocket loops, lateral pocket loops, twinned loops or accidentals.

Identification of any fingerprint is made by comparison of many details of characteristics, which occur throughout the ridge areas and by the sequence in which these characteristics occur, but not by comparing the patterns. The characteristics may take the form of ridge endings, bifurcations, lake formations or island formations. In practice, 16-20 points of fine comparison are accepted as proof of identity. The patterns are not inherited and paternity cannot be proved through fingerprints patterns. The details of these can be accurately teleprinted. Palm and footprints also provide similar material.

Exemplar prints: An exemplar print or known as prints, is the name given to fingerprints deliberately collected from a subject, whether for purposes of enrolment in a system or when under arrest for a suspected criminal arrests, a set of exemplar prints will normally include one print taken from each finger that has been rolled from one edge of the nail to the other, plain (or slap) impressions of each of four fingers of each hand, and plain impression of each thumb. Exemplar prints can be collected using live scan or by using ink on paper cards[1].

Latent prints[1]

Although the word latent means hidden or invisible, in modern usage for forensic science the term latent prints means any chance or accidental impression left by friction of epidermal ridges of skin on a surface, regardless of whether it is visible or invisible at the time of deposition. Electronic, chemical and physical invisible latent print residues, whether they are form natural sweat of the skin or from containment, such as motor oil, blood, ink, paint or some other form of dirt.

Latent prints may exhibit only a small portion of the surface of a finger, and this may be smudged, distorted, overlapped by other prints from the same or from different individuals or any or all of thesein combination. For this reason, latent prints usually present an "inevitable source of error in making comparisons", as they generally "contain less clarity, less content, and less undistorted information than a fingerprint taken under controlled conditions, and much less detail compared to the actual patterns of ridges and grooves of a finger.[1]

Patent prints [1]

Patent prints are chance friction ridge impressions, which are obvious to thehuman eye and which have been caused by the transfer of foreign material from a finger onto a surface. Some of obvious examples would be impression from flour and wet clay. Because they are already visible and have no need for enhancement, they are generally photographed rather than being lifted in the way the latent prints are. An attempt preserve the actual print is always made for later presentation in court, and there are many techniques used to do this. Patent prints can be left on a surface by materials such as ink, dirt or blood.[1]

Plastic prints[1]

The plastic print is an impression made on a soft surface, such as soap, cheese, etc. a plastic print is a friction ridge impression left in a material that retains the shape of the ridge detail. Although very few criminals would be careless enough to leave their prints in a lump of wet clay, this would make a perfect plastic print. Commonly encountered examples are melted candle wax; putty removed from the perimeter of windowpanes and thick grease deposits in car parts. Such prints are already visible and need no enhancement, but investigators must not overlook the potential that invisible latent prints deposited by accomplices may also be on such surfaces. After photographically recording such prints, attempts should be made to develop other non-plastic impressions deposited from sweat or other contaminates.[1]

The individuality of fingerprints[1]

The fingerprint patterns are distinctive and permanent in individuals. The fingerprint system is only guide to identify, which is unfailing in practice. The pattern is different even in identical twins and exhibit endless variation so that it has been speculated that there is one in 64 billion chances of two persons having identical fingerprints.

Mode of production [1]

Skin is covered by stream of sweat, and when the person is excited, the output of sweat increases. sweat contain about 99% water and 1% solids, which include salt, urea, fatty acids, formic acids, acetic acid , butyric acid , sometimes, a little albumin. The fingerprint may also contain oil exuded by the sebaceous glands, which is present on the fingertips through touching the face, neck hair, scalp, etc. if any part of finger is applied to a smooth surface; a greasy impression of its pattern is made on it.

Techniques of fingerprint[1]

The hands are washed, cleaned and dried, as otherwise the print will be blurred. Fingerprints are recorded on unglazed white paper using printers ink as follows: (1) a plain print is taken by applying ink to the tips of the fingers directly on paper; (2) the rolled fingerprint is taken by rolling the fingers on paper from outwards to inward in such a way as to obtain an impression of the whole tip burnt skin of the fingers, on healing shows its original pattern. In manual laborers working with lime, sand and cement, the ridge on the bulbs get unduly rubbed and become broken and indistinct. Ridge impressions get malformed if the quality of ink is poor, when the ink is too liquid and spreads into the depressions, if the digit is rolled often or pulled and when paper is placed upon an uneven or rough surface.

Fingerprints may be taken from almost any surface with which the finger comes in contact, including certain fabrics and human skin. A latent print may be developed by dusting the area with colored powders to provide a contrast, and its pattern is recorded by photography. It can also be examined by oblique lighting. The commonly used powder is **gray powder** (aluminum dust), but **white powders(lead carbonate or French chalk)** are used for dusting dark surfaces. Iodine vapors, and silicon nitrate solution are also used for developing fingerprints on paper. Wood and fabrics are developed by exposing it to the autoradiography method uses a high-energy beam of X-ray to irradiate the lead dust on fingers mark. The scanning electron microscope visualizes latent fingerprints on metal and glass.

Lifting of fingerprints

Fingerprints on large immovable hard surface is usually first developed, photographed and then adhesive surface of cellophane tape is pressed on the print, taken out gently and then it is pasted against a cardboard sheet for permanent preservation.

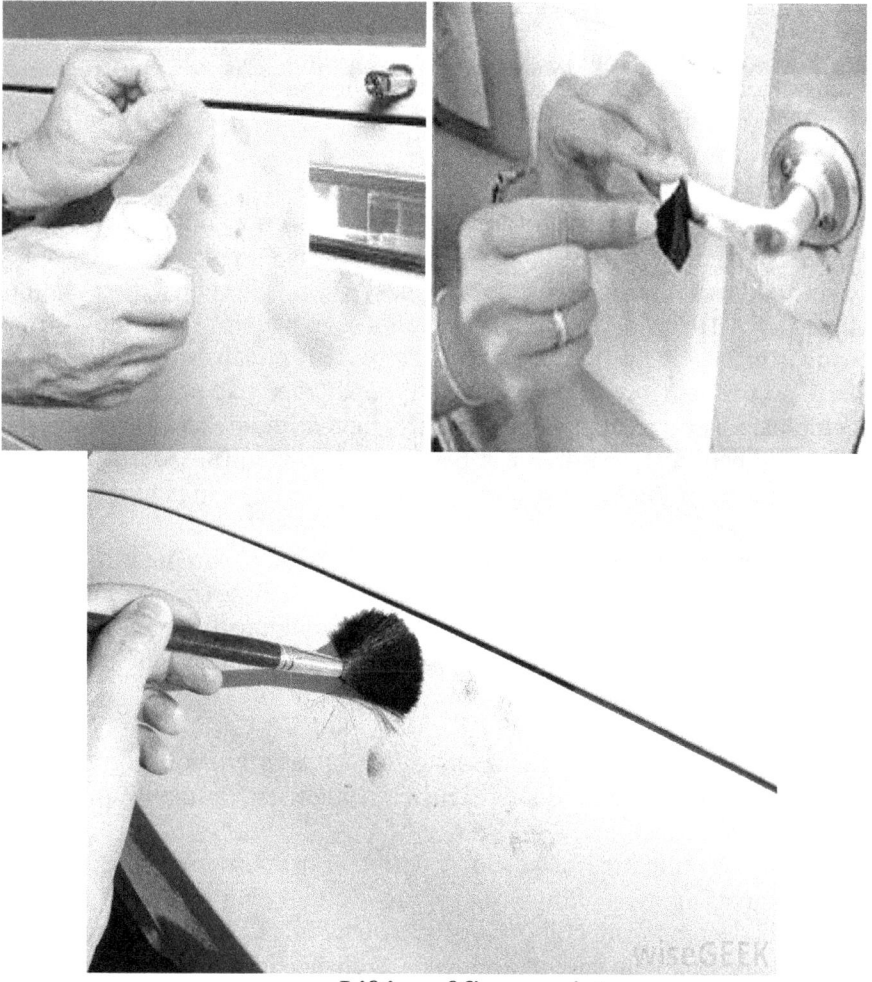

Lifting of finger prints

FINGERPRINTS IN DECOMPOSED BODIES[1, 4]

Ridges are present in both dermis and epidermis. In advanced putrefaction and in cases of drowning. The sin is frequently found loose like a glove. This should be removed preserved in formalin and used for impressions.

Prints can be obtained from the dermis after epidermis is lost. Histological sections up to a depth of 0.6mm from the surface of the skin give satisfactory fingerprints. In dead bodies, the palmar skin of the terminal phalanx of each finger should be removed separately from both hands, and after looking placed in separate containers containing 10% formalin, and sent to the fingerprint bureau, if it is not possible to take the prints. If the fingers areshriveled, they should be immersed in 20% acetic acid for 24-48 hours.[1, 4]

If the fingers are sodden, wrinkled or mummified, their outline can be made level by injecting liquid paraffin, or even formalin, within the tissues of the palmar aspects of the terminal phalanx of each finger.[1]

Persistence of impression at scene of crime: impressions may persist for years, if undisturbed by cleaning. Even outside the house, they may persist for weeks. On glazed paper, they persist more than 3 years.[1]

Mutilation of fingerprints [1]

Criminals sometimes attempt to mutilate the pattern of self-inflicted wounds or burns, application of corrosives or erosion against hard surfaces, but the prints are not destroyed unless the true skin is completely destroyed. They produce additional characteristics. In most cases of celiac disease, there is moderate epidermal ridge atrophy and even loss of pattern. Incomplete atrophy of the ridges is usually seen in dermatitis. Permanent impairment of the fingerprint pattern occurs in leprosy, electric injury and after exposure to radiation. In infantile paralysis, rickets and acromegaly, though the pattern is not altered; but the distance between the ridges can be changed. Fingerprints are better protected than other parts of the body, e.g. in case of burns. They are bent inwards against the palm of the hand.

Computerization: fingerprint reader (FINDER) is a computerized automatic fingerprint reading system, which can record each fingerprint datum in a half second. Prints of eight fingers are recorded, excluding little fingers. The light reflected from a fingerprint can be measured and converted to digital data, which is classified, codified and stored in the computer.[1, 4]

Medicolegal importance

➢ The recognition of impressions left at a scene of a crime, e.g. on weapons, furniture, doors, utensils, clothes, etc., establish the identity of the criminal.

➢ The identification of suicides, deserters, persons suffering from loss of memory or those dead or unconscious after being involved in an accident and decomposing bodies can be made by this technique.

➢ Identification in case of accidental exchange of newborn infants.

➢ The prevention of impersonation.

➢ To maintain identity records.

In criminals, impressions of all the 10 fingers are taken, but for civil purposes, only the left thumb impression is taken.

POROSCOPY[1]

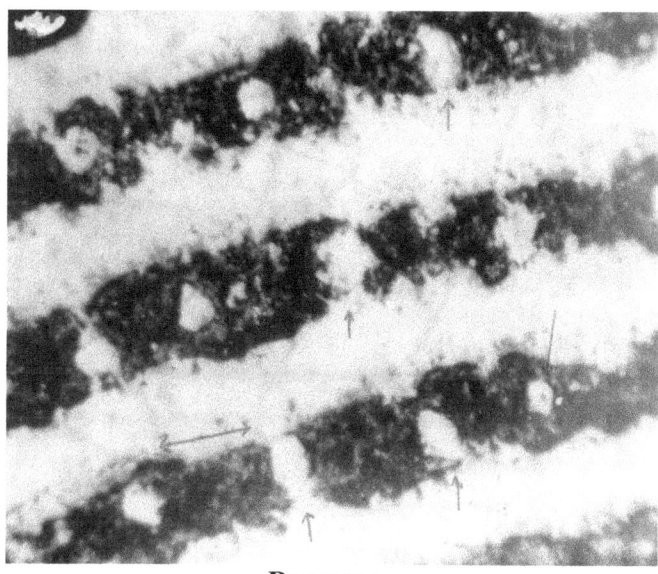

Poroscopy

The method was discovered and developed by Edmond locard in 1912. The ridges on fingers and hands are studded with microscopic pores, formed by mouths of ducts of subepidermal sweat glands. Each arm of a ridge contains 9-18 pores. These pores are permanent and unchanged during life and vary in size, shape, position, extent and number over a given length of ridge in each individual. This method of examining pores is called poroscopy and is useful when only fragments of fingerprints are available.

Palm prints[1]

It may identity a person, if his hands were moist with blood or fluids. A palm print refers to an image acquired of the palm region of the hand. It can be either an online image, i.e. taken by a scanner, or CCD device or offline image where the image is taken with ink and paper. It is an extension of the fingerprint system, which records and matches images of the entire palm.

FOOTPRINTS (PODOGRAM) [1]

The skin pattern of toes and heels areas distinct and permanent as those of the fingers, footprints of newborn infants are used in some maternity hospitals to prevent exchange or substitution of infants.

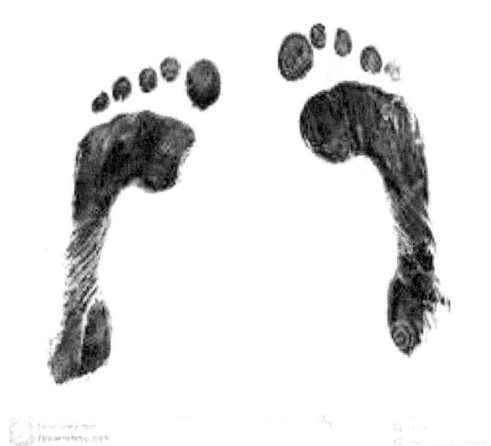 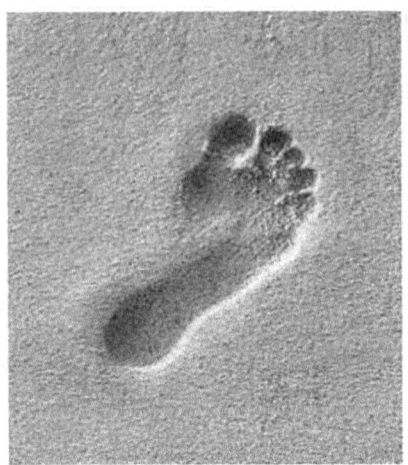

Foot prints

A fresh footprint of a suspected person is taken and compared with the original any peculiarities in the foot, such as a flat foot, supernumerary toes, scars or callosities are likely to be found in the footprint. In case of bookmark, the pattern and arrangement of nails or holes in the sole may be useful. A footprint produced by walking is usually larger than one produced by standing. The imprint on soft loose material like sand is smaller than the foot, and the imprint produced on mud or clay is larger.

A footmark expert may identify a shoe with a mark made at the scene of crime and by general examination may find out the number of persons involve there and their actual movements at the scene and their point of entry. Individual impressions, especially in yielding soil, will indicate the shoe size and approximate weight of the person and any peculiarity of gait. A partial footmark may be quite sufficient to positively identify a shoe. Footmarks are recorded by photography; casts or lifting or by combination. Casts can only be taken when there is a footmark in depth. As they are three dimensional, they can easily be compared with the suspects shoe's even by lay persons.[1]

Foot prints are helpful in

- Identification in relation to chance footprints found at the scene of crime,
- To prevent deliberate or accidental substitution of babies in maternity hospitals.

Footprints record are maintained for all air force flying personnel in most countries since feet often resist destruction by aircraft accident, fires, etc.[2]

LIP PRINTS (CHEILOSCOPY)[1]
Definition

It is the study of wrinkles and cracks of lips that has specific individual characters. They are useful in personal identification.

History

Identification using lip print was first performed in the 1950s and was the subject of much research in the 1960s and 70s, leading to the acceptance of this technique as evidence in the criminal justice system.

Features

Previous research has focused on identifying lip print types or on methods of obtaining hidden lip print types or on methods of obtaining hidden lip print left at the crime scene. Lip prints are divided into **six different patterns**vertical, partial straight, branched, intersected, and reticular, and undifferentiated patterns. Minor differences can be noted between the right and the left and upper and lower lips.[1]

1. short vertical lines

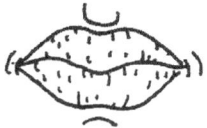

2. long vertical lines

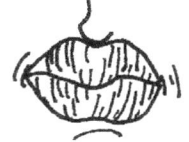

3. rectangular lines that may crisscross

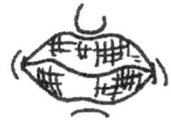

4. lines that form diamond patterns

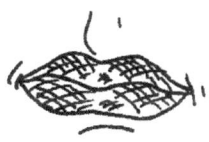

5. branching lines like those in a plant root

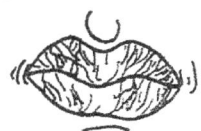

Different pattern of lip prints

SUPERIMPOSITION [1,2]

Superimpositionis the technique applied to determine whether the skull is that of the person in the photograph. A recent photograph is better. The photograph of lateral and semi-lateral view of face can also be used.[1,2]

Technique

If the negative of the photograph is not available, negative of the available photograph is prepared by recopying it. The photograph is enlargedto natural size from the presence of some standard thing in the photograph of the missing person to indicate the scale. The negative is placed under the ground glass of camera and salient features of the face are marked out carefully on the glass. The soft parts are removed from the skull. A comparison can be made even in the absence of the lower jaw. The skull is mounted on an appropriate skull rest to align it as accurately as possible with the outline of the head on the ground glass in the corresponding portrait, making due allowance for the tissues covering the bone. The distance of the camera is allowed is adjusted so that the one-inch scale on the ground glass of the camera is exactly equal to the scale on the skull. This, when photographed, gives a life sized negative of the photographs and the skull are superimposed by aligning the characteristic points in the negatives.[1, 2]

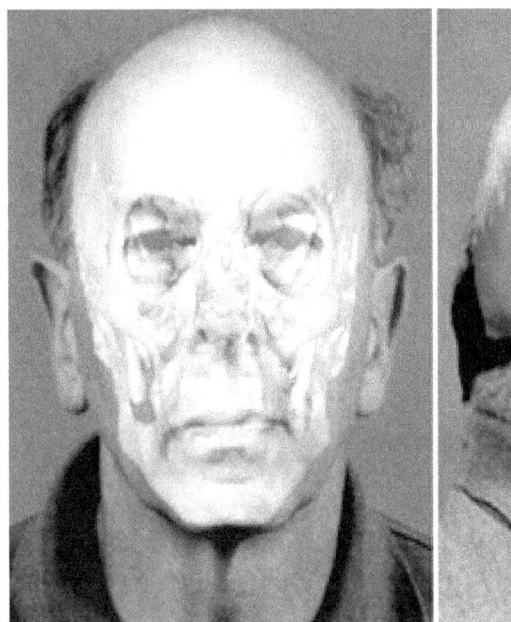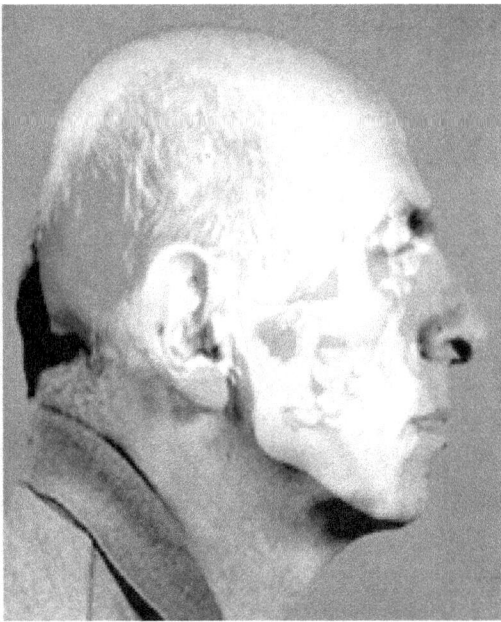

Superimposition

Comparison points
- The eyes within the orbital plates, with the two pairs of canthuses properly aligned
- The nasion
- The prosthion in the central line.
- The nasal spine in the center which is a little above the tip of the nose.
- The lower border of the nose
- The lower border of the upper jaw, i.e. below the tip of the nose.
- The zygomos below the eyes
- Supraorbital ridges
- Angle of the jaw
- External auditory meatus
- Teeth

The two superimposed negatives are then photographed on bromide paper. The resulting photograph brings out the points of similarity or dissimilarity between the photograph and the skull. The superimposition is correct if the outlines and the size of the skull accurately correspond to the face in the photograph. A clear effect of the superimposed area can be obtained by combining the negative of the skull with the positive of portrait. For this, positive and negative of the skull are rephotographed on X-ray film, thus producing a transparent positive of the skull. Finally, the two films are bound together in register and thus superimposed; they are then rephotographed on X-ray film by transmitted light.

Opinion: the test is of a more negative value because it can definitely be stated that the skull and the photograph are not those of the same person. If they tally, it can only be stated that the skull could be that of the person in the photograph, because of the possibility that another skull of that size and contour may tally with the photograph.

Disadvantages: even a slight variation in the magnification of the photograph or change in angulations of skull can lead to major differences resulting in mismatch. The process is laborious and time consuming.

Computer-assisted skull identification using video superimposition

The skull is mounted on an adjustable support allowing movement in three planes.

The photograph is also mounted similarly. A colored video camera is aligned at right angles to the photograph and a second camera is aligned to the skull. The individual video signals from each camera are fed into a vision mixer. By this, superimposition and negative simulation can be done. In cases where sufficient anterior teeth remain on the cranium and a photograph showing suspected decreased smiling is available, image superimposition can be done. Digital image manipulation technique is better.

This system consists of two main units, namely a video superimposition system and a computer-assisted skull identification system. The video superimposition system comprised of the following five parts: a skull-positioning box having a monochrome CCD camera, a photo-stand having a color CCD camera, a video image mixing device, a TV monitor and a videotape recorder. The computer-assisted skull identification system is composed of a host computer including original application software, a film recorder and a color printer. After the determination of the orientation and size of the skull to those of the facial photograph images are digitized and stored within the computer, and then both digitized images are superimposed on the monitor.

For the assessment of anatomical consistency between the digitized skull and face, the distance between the landmarks and the thickness of soft tissue of the anthropometrical points are semi-automatically measured on the monitor. The wipe images facilitate the comparison of positional relationships between the digitized skull and face.

The software includes the polynomial functions and Fourier harmonic analysis for evaluating the march of the outline such as the forehead and mandibular line in both the digitized images.

DEFORMITIES AND BIRTHMARKS

They may be congenital or acquired. Congenital deformities, such as talipes, polydactylism, web-fingers or toes, undescended testicles, harelip, cleft palate etc., are frequently treated surgically and are, therefore, losing some of their past importance. Old amputations, spinal defects, old fractures and deformities of the bones and nails, either from injuries or disease and surgical prostheses, such as implanted artificial heart valves, plates in the skull etc., should be described.

Birthmarks

A birthmark is a skin marking that ispresent at birth. Birthmark includes cafe-au-lait spots, moles (caused by excess skin pigment cells) and Mongolian spots. Birthmarks are usually caused by overgrowth of blood vessels, melanocytes, smooth muscle, fat, fibroblasts, or keratinocytes.[1]

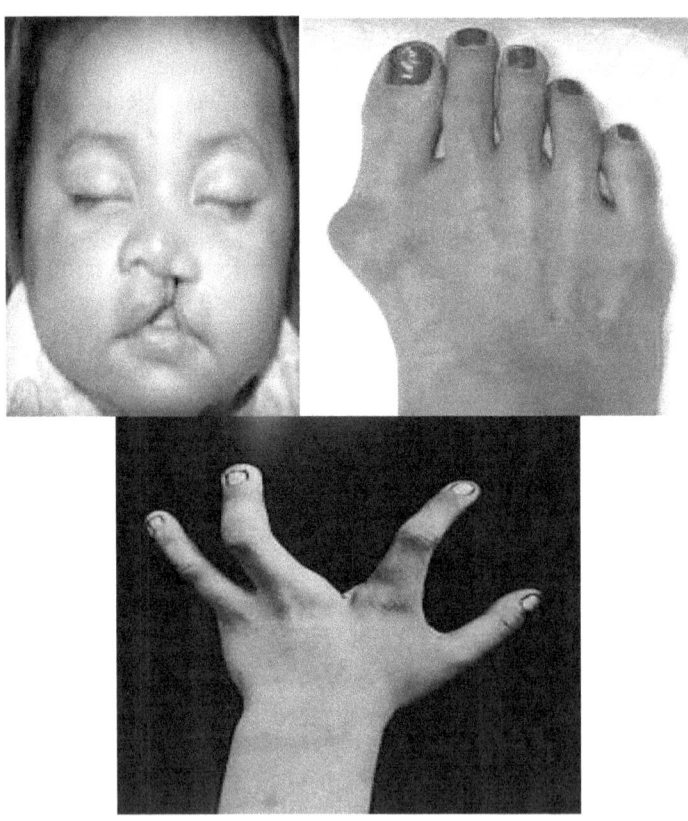

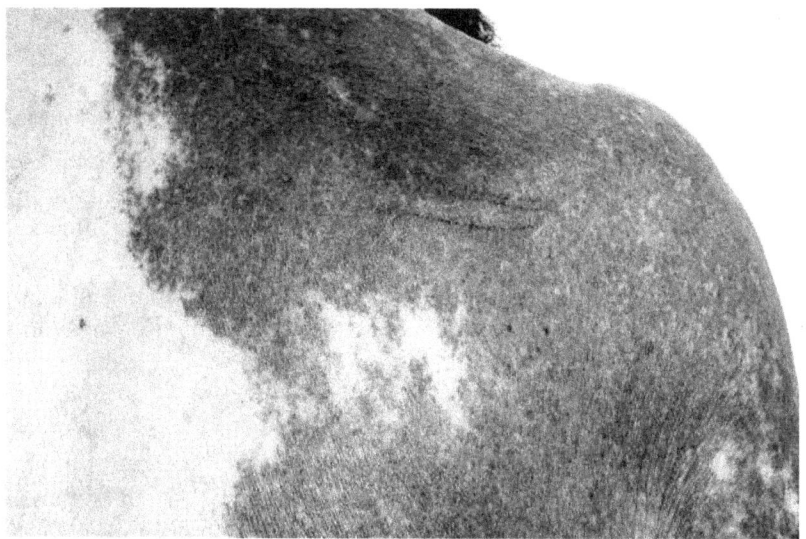
Deformities and birthmark

Moles are usually round, brown or black, raised or flat with or without hair. The size and exact anatomical position should be noted. A Mongolian spot (congenital marks) appear as dark blue or violet, single or multiple maculae in the lumbosacral region in some young children of Asiatic and African origin.[3]

SCARS

A scar is the result of are pair mechanism to an injury involving the dermis of the skin. These are simply the fibrous tissues covered by epithelium without hair follicles, pigments or sweat glands, produced from the healing of a wound. Injury to the dermis produces a scar, while superficial injuries involving only the epidermis do not produce a scar. Scars are permanent.[1]

Examination

Examination of scar is done in good light and description should include their number, site, size and shape, the level it bears to the body surface, fixed or free, smoothness or irregularity of the surface, color and the presence or absence of the glistening and tenderness. The condition of the ends, whether tapering or not, and the probable direction of original wound should be determined. The application of heart, filtered ultraviolet light or surface friction, marks faint scars readily visible. A magnifying glass is very useful. Suspected scars in the dead body can be proved by microscopy, by a section stained to show the elastic tissue, which is absent in a scar. Elastic tissue is present in striae gravidarum.

Characters

The shape of the scars may indicate the type of injury which produced them
  - Incised wounds produce linear scar. If healing is secondary, the scar is wider and thicker in the center than in the periphery.
  - Scars from lacerated wounds are firmer, irregular, more prominent and are attached to the deeper tissues.

- Stab wound due to knife-blade produces oval, elliptical, triangular or irregular scars, which are depressed but may be elevated due to keloid formation.
- A bullet wound causes a circular depressed scar.
- Scars from scalds are spotted in appearance, tend to be continuous, often run downwards and show evidence of splashing about the main injury.
- Scars due to corrosive acids, burns or radiation are irregular and keloid may develop in the scar tissue.
- Vaccination scars are circular or oval flat or slight depressed(figure)
- Many skin diseases, like smallpox and syphilis, cause multiple scars on the skin.

Growth

A scar produced in childhood, grows in size with the natural development of the individual, especially if situated on the chest or limbs.

A keloid also known as **keloidal scar**, is a type of scar, which depending on its maturity, is composed mainly of collagen. It results of an overgrowth of granulation tissue (collagen type III) at the site of a healed skin injury, which is then slowly replaced by collagen type 1. Keloids are firm, rubbery lesions or shiny, fibrous nodules and can vary in color from pink to flesh-colored or red to dark brown (figure).

Age of scars

Freshly formed scar appears reddish or bluish and is tender and soft. These features are appreciated for about a couple of weeks. Due to gradual decrease in the vascularity, it is pale but is still tender and soft up to a couple of months. Then the scars contracts, but still is little tender and soft. The age of such scar is between 2 to 6 months. As the scar contracts further, it becomes tough, white and glistening. Such scar is probably not less than 6 months old. After this, there is no further change.

Erasure:

The scar can be erased by excision and skin grafting or suture of the edges of the excised area. This results in a scar, which is less clearly seen.

Medicolegal importance

- They form important marks for identification of a person.
- The age of the scar is important in a criminal offence. If the age of a wound criminal offence. If the age of a wound corresponds with the date of the attack, it may have value in circumstantial evidence.
- The shape of the scar may indicate the nature of weapon or agent that caused the injury.
- The person may be disfigured due to scars, or contracture around a joint produced by scar may restrict the movement and function of the joint, making it a grievous hurt.
- Linea albicantes may indicate previous pregnancy.
- The accused may attribute scars of wounds to disease or therapeutic procedures.

➢ To charge an enemy with assault, a person may claim that scars due to disease are those of wounds.[1]

TATTOO MARKS[1]

The word 'tattoo' comes from Polynesian 'tatau' meaning to 'mark'. Tattoo marks are a good identification marks for both living and dead, and provide a wide range of information about the person having them. Tattoo marks are designs (figure) made by multiple small puncture wounds in the skin through needles or similar penetrating tools dipped in a coloring dye. The permanency of tattoo marks depends upon the type of dye used, the depth of its penetration and the part of body tattooed.

The dyes commonly used are Indian ink, carbon (black) cinnabar or vermilion (red), chromium (green), indigo, cobalt, Prussian blue and ultra marine (blue). Techniques and dyes vary from country to country. Tattooing may be done mechanically on by electrical device.

Most of the marks are found on the arm, forearm and chest, but may be present on any part of the body. The most permanent pictures are made when the dye penetrates the dermis. If the dye is deposited in the deeper layer of the dermis, it will be removed by phagocytes. Tattoos slowly become fainter and certain pigments, such as vermilion and ultramarine may disappear after about 10 years. The rate of fading depends not only on the composition of the pigment but also on the depth to which it penetrates the skin and the site, which is tattooed: parts protected by clothing retain the design for longer period than the exposed part of the body.

Due to constant friction, tattoos on the hands disappear early. A faded tattoo mark becomes visible by the use of ultraviolet lamp or rubbing the part and examining with magnifying lens. Infrared photography marks old tattoos readily visible. The marks are recognized even in decomposed bodies when the epidermis is removed. Lymph nodes near a tattoo mark show a deposit of a pigment.[1]

Complications

Tattooing can lead to septic inflammation, erysipelas, abscess and gangrene. Syphilis, AIDS, leprosy and tuberculosis may occur due to sharing of the needle.

Erasures

1) Surgical methods:
   i.   Complete excision and skin grafting
   ii. Production of burn by means of red hot iron,
   iii. Scarification and,
   iv. Carbon dioxide snow.
2) Electrolysis.
3) Caustic substances remove pigment by producing inflammatory reaction and a superficial scar, e.g. mixture of papain in glycerin, zinc chloride and tannic acid.
4) Laser beam: by exposure to laser beams, the particles of the dye get vaporized and are expelled from the tissues in gaseous form

5) Confluent smallpox and, sometimes, chronic eczema in children can obliterate tattoo marks.

Medicolegal importance

- ➢ Positive identification can be made by tattoo alone, if there is a large number of tattoos, initials and dates, regimental details, identity numerals, one's own name, etc.
- ➢ Religion designs of cross or Christ(in Christians) and Hanuman, Lord Krishna (in Hindus) may provide religions.
- ➢ Tattoos may also represent someone's social status.
- ➢ The distribution of tattooing and the nature of designs and figures may indicate a particular country or region.
- ➢ The presence of indecent figure points to definite perversion in the individual.
- ➢ They reflect travel, history, war, occupation, sex interest, etc.
- ➢ Drugs addicts may tattoo front of elbow or wrist to conceal needle puncture marks.
- ➢ Race: extensive tattooing of the chest and limbs is common among the Japanese.
- ➢ Profession, some criminal gangs have certain specific emblems of tattoo marks. Some occupations, e.g. coal miners leave visible tattoo marks on the hand and face from the material handled by the workers. Political convictions like sword and sickle, cow and calf.
- ➢ Behavioral characteristics like erotic tattoos of the sexual fanatic, blue bird design on the extensor surface of the web of the thumb of homosexuals, number 13 inside the lower lip of drug pushers, addict type of tattoo marks to conceal injection sites, etc.[1]

DISEASE, WOUNDS AND STAINS[1]
DISEASE

The finding of a disease, e.g. gall stones, renal stones, calcified leiomyoma, silicosis, asbestosis, and congenital anomalies, like horseshoe kidney, is helpful in identification of an individual. The unidentified body should be checked for amputations, body deformities, pacemakers , implanted heart valves, enlarged joints of the fingers due to arthritis, immovable joints due to disease, bowed legs and curvature of the spine. X-rays will show the presence of healed fracture, metal pins, plates or screw used in treating fractures. Commonly found missing organs at autopsy are tonsils, appendix, gallbladder , kidney, prostate, uterus and ovaries. Surgical scars may indicate hernia repair, circumcision or an operation upon the thyroid gland

WOUNDS[1]

Sometimes, the presence of wounds on the body may assist in connecting a suspected criminal with a given crime, e.g. a piece of skin adherent to a window glass may correspond with the wound on the thief or rupture of frenum of penis may be present ina person accused of rape. Dust, sand, etc. may be recovered from wounds and identified.

STAINS[1]

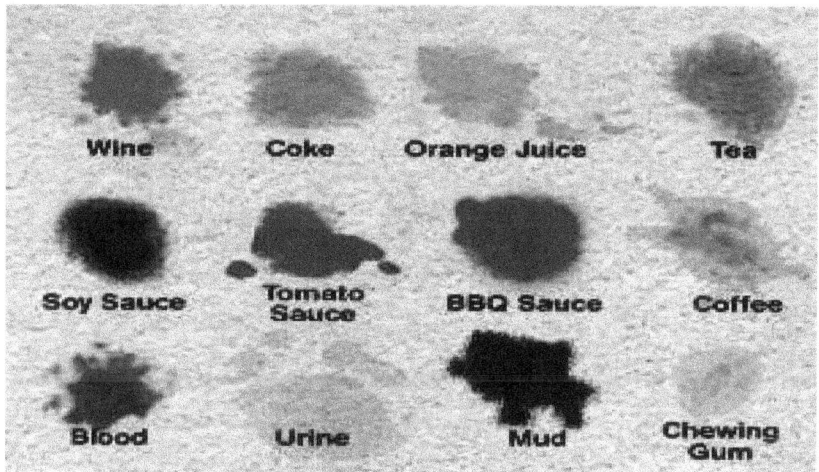

Stains found on body or clothing of the accused and the victim may be the same may be derived from the walls, doors, furniture etc. at the scene of crime.[1]

Occupational stigmata[1, 4]

Occupational marks are the characteristics that result from adaptation to work. Distinctive marks of occupation have decreased in incidence and importance but still some of these can be useful for identification. They may be recent and temporary, and permanent marks. [1, 4]

Recent and temporary

They include paint spots or painters, grease on engineers and mechanics, flour on bakers and millers and dyes on dye workers. A microscopic examination of dust and debris on clothing in the pocket, under the fingernails and in the ear wax is important in identification of unknown bodies. They may also connect the body with a specific place where a crime was committed.

Permanent

A callosity is seen on the outer side of the distal phalanx of the middle finger of the right hand of a clerk. This is really seen these days thickening of the palmar skin of fingers are seen on the right hands of butchers. Manual laborer show horny and rough hands. Tailors have marks of needle punctures on their left index finger. Certain occupations may change the colour of the hair, e.g. hair of copper smelters may be greenish while that of indigo workers and cobalt miners are bluish. Coal miners have 'blue scars' on the face and arms due to coal dust contamination of small lacerations, steel workers usually have multiple small scars from metal burns. Workers in chemical and photography usually have discoloured, distorted fingernails. Carpenters have callosities on the thumb and index finger,on the palms and one shoulder is usually higher than the other. The violinist has hardened tips on the fingers of the left hand.

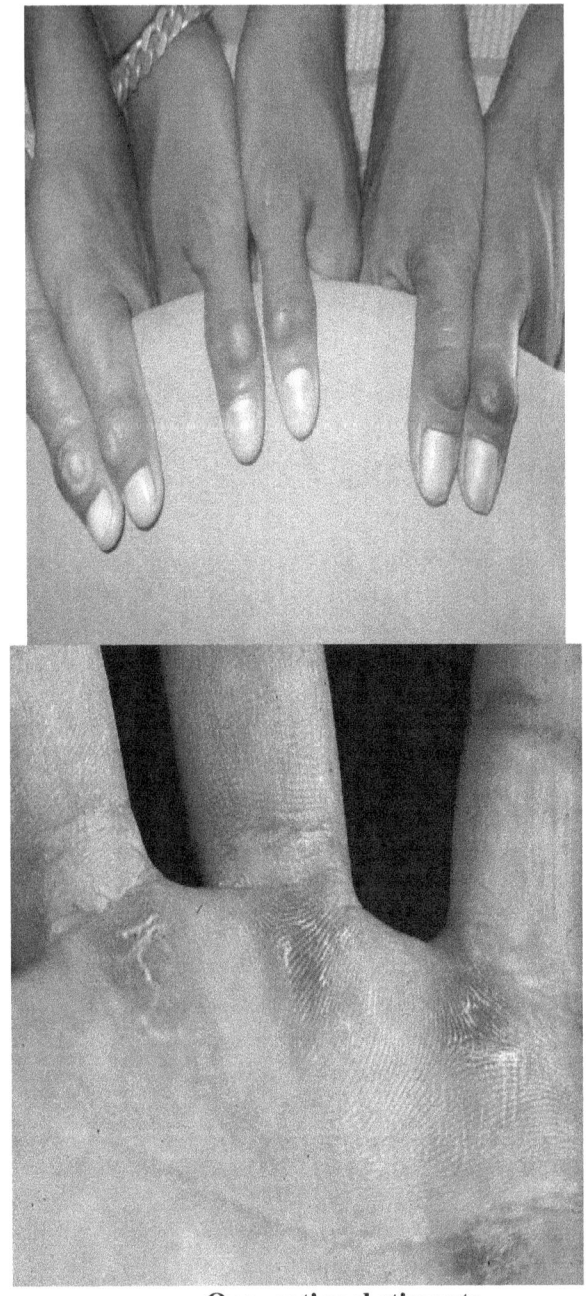

Occupational stigmata

COMLEXION AND FEATURES[1]

Complexion may be fair, white coloured, dark brown, pale brown, pale yellow. Details of the features regarding eyes, hair, nose, ears, eyebrows, lips, chin and teeth should benoted. The features may change considerably from disease or even from worries over a long duration.

Shape of mouth, nose, ear, eyebrows, beard and moustache are the important points, which help in identity establishment. Any irregularities of teeth, artificial teeth, etc. are also helpful in this event. Few persons can cleverly alter their features by changing their face expression. Expression is altered after death.

CLOTHES AND ORNAMENTS

The clothing, from the texture and value may indicate the social status to a certain extent. Any variety of uniform is very valuable for identification. Clothing may also indicate the occupation. The examination of clothing and personal effects is helpful in the identification of victims in mass disaster, such as fires, explosions and aircraft crashes. A detailed description of the size , colour, condition and type of garment and a record of laundry marks , name tags and labels of tailors should be given. Photograph and examination for invisible laundry marks by ultra violet light are useful, the clothing may contain keys, letters, bank books, visiting cards, license or other documents which may give a clue to the name and address of the individual. Other personal effects like watches, rings, keys, belt buckles, etc. may be engraved with initials, name or dates. Eye glasses may also be helpful. A criminal may interchange his identity with that of another person, clothing and personal effects. Bullet holes, tears, cut or tyre marks found on clothing may give information regarding the cause and manner of death. The design of ornaments varies from region to region.

General cleanliness of the person and the state of the teeth, hands, feet, give some idea of social status. If shoes are worn, the epidermis of the souls of the feet is thin and smooth without any fissures and cracks.

HAIR
HUMAN HAIR

Study of hair is known as trichology. In most of the human hair, there are three well defined layers as follows:

a) Cuticle : this the outer layer and consist of thin non pigmented scales.

b) Cortex : this the middle layer comprising of longitudinally arranged, elongated cells without nuclei.

c) Medulla : within these cells, there will be granules of pigment. This is the innermost layer composed of keratinized remains of the cell. It may be narrow, absent, fragmented or discontinuous.

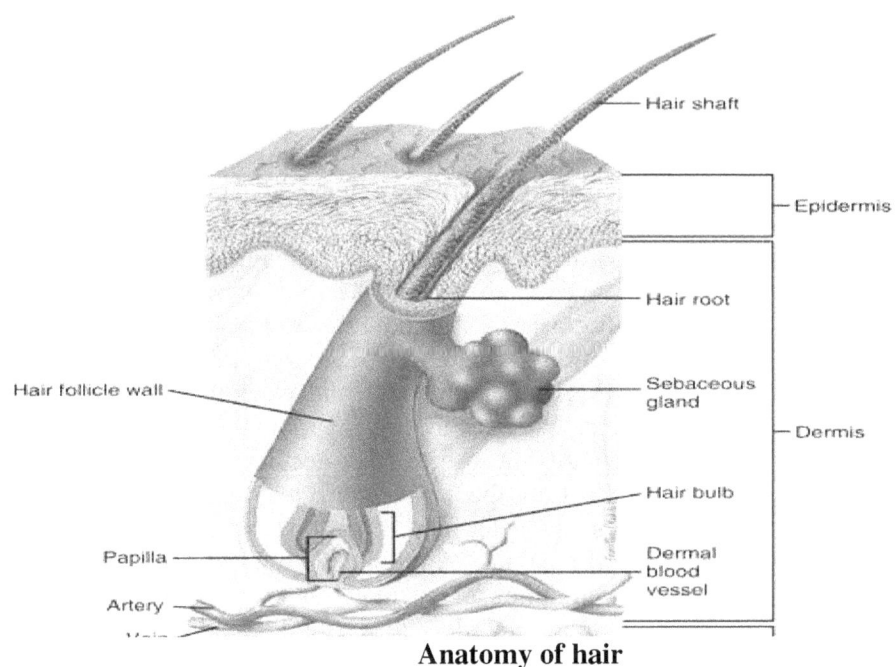

Anatomy of hair

Labels: Hair shaft, Epidermis, Hair root, Sebaceous gland, Dermis, Hair bulb, Dermal blood vessel, Hair follicle wall, Papilla, Artery

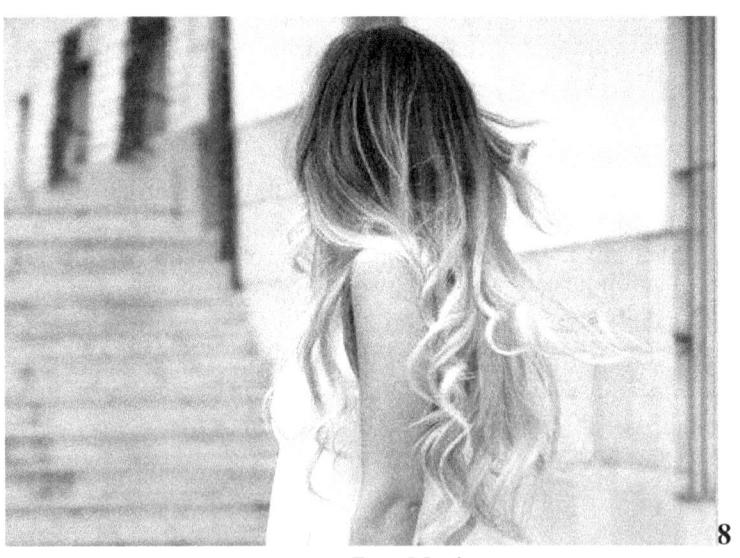

Dyed hair

FIBRES[1]

      Cloth fibers often seen at the site of crime or on a suspect. In some cases, small piece of cloth may be found. The police may find a matching piece of cloth whose torn edge will fit the torn edge of the first piece. such a match is called jigsaw fit. There are some simple test, which help greatly in distinguishing fabrics, the most common being the burning test and chemical test. The fibers may be of cotton, linen, jute, silk etc. they may resemble hair . each fiber has different morphological features.

LINEN FIBRES

Made from fibers of the flax plant, the linum usitatissimum fiber is linear, jointed, segmented with swelling like bamboo. Fibers usually run in bundles.

SILK FIBERS

It is natural protein fiber, some form of which can be woven into textiles. The shimmering appearance of the silk is due to triangular prison like structure. Which allow silk cloth to refract incoming light at different angles, thus producing different colours.fibers are long, clear, regular, cylindrical, retractile threads without any cell with any twisting or joints or swelling.

COTTON FIBER

Is soft, fluffy staple fiber. It is fairly uniform in width, flattened, twisted, tube like bands with thickened edges and blunt pointed end.[1, 4]

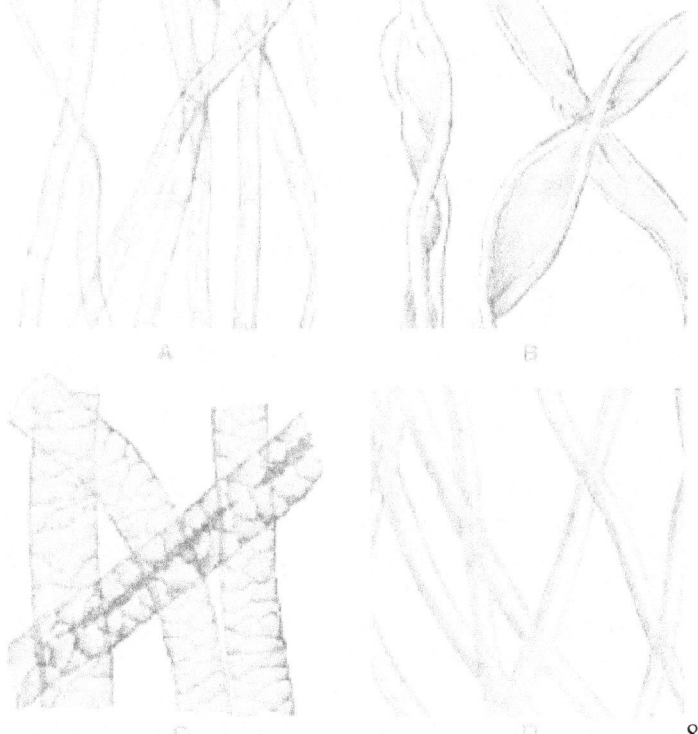

8

Magnified fibers of linen, cottonwool and silk

77

DIFFERENCE BETWEEN HUMAN AND ANIMAL HAIR[1]

TRAIT	HUMAN HAIR	ANIMAL HAIR
General	Fine and thin	Coarse and thick
Cuticle	Scales short, broad thin, irregularly annular	Scales large and has step like wavy projection.
Cortex	Thick, 4-10 times as broad as medulla	Thin, twice as broad as medulla
Medulla	Narrow non-continuous, fragmented	Continuous and wider
Pigment	Evenly distributed	Mostly near medulla
Precipitin test	Specific for human	Specific for animal
Medullary index	<0.3	>0.5

Identification of hair from different part of the body

Scalp hair is usually soft and tappers gradually from the root of the tip. The beard and moustache are thicker than other parts of the body. The hair on the chest, axilla and pubic region is short, stout, and curly. There may be split ends in hair from axillary and pubic region. Hair of eyebrow, eyelash and nostril are stiff, thick and taper to a point. The hair from other parts of the body is fine, short and does not show pigment cells in the cortex.[1]

Identification of hair in different sex

Male hair is usually thicker, coarser and darker. In human scalp hair, the barr bodies are found in hair follicles in about 30% females and 6% males. Presence of certain hair like that from beard and moustache makes the sex determination easier.

Atebrin stained hair roots under fluorescent microscope is an easy, quick and efficient method for accurate counting of Barr bodies in females, Y bodies in males and simultaneously both types of bodies in Klinefelter's patients. Refractive index appears to be one of the most significant differences between male and female hair.

Identification of hair in different ages

The age can be determined by hair with vary wide limits. Root of hair from children will dissolve rapidly in a solution of caustic potash, but in elderly people, roots will resist the treatment. Fetus and newborn child have fine, soft, non-pigmented and non-medullated hair called as *lanugo hair*. This lanugo hair is replaced by coarser, pigmented and medullated hair, which has more complex scale pattern.

The diameter of hair increases from childhood to adult age group: 0.024mm in new born child, 0.053mm at 15 years and 0.07mm in adults. At puberty, the axillary and pubic hairs grow which is fine, soft and curly and later become coarse and pigmented.Maximum pigmentation is seen in adult hair. Grey hair usually appears after 40 years

Hair is altered by dyeing, bleaching and diseases. Bleached hair is brittle, dry and straw yellow. Colored hair is rough, brittle and lusterless and color is not uniformly seen. Color of hair is different from other parts of the body. The time of color last applied can be known by measuring the uncolored part at the base which has grown after color application. The scalp hair grows at a rate of 2-3mm a week. Any metal present in the paint can be found out by chemical examination of hair. Dyed hair shows fluorescence and ultra violet light.

If the hair bulb is present, ABO blood group can be determined from single hair from any part of the body by modified absorption elusion method. The distribution and concentration of trace elements along shaft of the hair varies as the hair grows. The color of hair may vary with diseases it is lighter in malnutrition ulcerative colitis and kwashiorkor. This may become normal with restoration of health. Color of hair becomes green from copper, yellow from picricacid and cobalt poisoning.

Medicolegal questions

> ## Is the hair identical to that of suspect?

It can be said that the hair could have come from particular person by careful examination of debris, grease, etc. adherent to hair. Factors, which help in individualization:

a) ABO blood grouping can be done in a single hair from any part by modified absorption elusion technique with 100% accuracy.
b) Isozyme typing i.e., PGM, RGD, AK, GLO, etc.
c) Identification of trace elements by neuron activation analysis.
d) Evidence of disease.
e) Evidence of application of dyes, henna etc.

> ## Did the hair fall was naturally or forcibly removed?

The base must be examined for the presence of the root. In a naturally fallen hair, the root will be distorted and atrophied without sheath.If the hair is forcibly pulled out, hair will be larger and the sheath will be rupture.

> ## What is the cause if injury?

The tip of the hair is pointed and non-medullated if hair has not been cut, but repeated injury to tip damages the cuticle resulting in splitting and fraying of the cortex. A sharp weapon produces a uniform cut surface while a blow with blunt object crushes the shaft with flattening and splitting. Hair may get singed due to burn and firearm injury, there the hair is swollen, black, fragile, twisted or curled has a peculiar odor and may show deposition of carbon.

Medicolegal importance of hair and fiber

> Hair is valuable trace element in crime investigation as it remains on clothes, body and on weapons for a long time. It can be a connecting link between the weapon or even the accused and the victim of an assault. In sexual offences like rape, sodomy, the pubic hair of the accused may be found on the victim and vice versa. In bestiality, animal hair may be found on the body of the clothing of the accused or his hair may be found on the genitals of animal. The vehicle responsible for producing injuries in accidents can be identified by presence of hair on the vehicle.

Examination of the stains on the hair can be useful to indicate the nature of assault seminal stains in sexual offences, mud stains in struggle and blood stains in injuries.

- By observing the injuries to hair and hair bulb, the nature of weapon can be made out.
- Hair becomes useful in identification in the presence of some peculiarity like dying and bleaching.
- By growth of hair on different parts of the body, age of the person can be determined.
- By distribution, texture and barr bodies, sex of a person can be determined.
- Singeing of hair indicates burns or firearm injury (close range).
- Hair is useful in differentiating burns from scalds.
- The absorbent property of hair makes its examination important in cases of arsenic poisoning. Hair picks up the poison from the bloodstream, and it is possible to work out the approximate strength and frequency of the dosage by analysis.
- Time since death may be determined from of hair on face. Head hair grows at an average weekly rate of about 2.5mm, beard grows faster and body hair slower growth ceases at death, but as the skin shrinks, hair, especially the beard, becomes more prominent, giving rise to murder myth that hair grows after death.
- Hair can be used in helping to reconstruct events.
  Collection of hair and fibers can indicate contact with surfaces or individuals and so where individuals have been.
- Examination of the root structure can indicate whether hair has fallen out or been forcefully removed, indicating struggle.
- Hair can alsobe used to assist identification through DNA analysis. If some root structure is present, standard DNA profiling can be used. Even if you only have the shaft mitochondrial DNA testing can be tried.[1]

Miscellaneous
HAND WRITING (CALLIGRAPHY)

Handwriting of every individual is characteristic, especially if it is written rapidly, but it may be disguised or of forged. Mantle and nervous disease and rheumatism may alter the character of handwriting. Evidence of handwriting experts is opinion evidence, but it is not conclusive. [1-4,9]

SPEECH AND VOICE

Certain peculiarity of speech, e.g. stammering, stuttering, lisping and nasal twang, become more evident when the individual is excitedly should be noted. Speech is a; so affected by nervous disease. It is too risky to recognize a person from the voice alone it is possible for a person to alter his voice at a will. No two voices are really alike acoustic "spectrogram "characteristic of the speaker can be produced by utterance of a single syllable plotted on time baseline. This can be utilized in trapping anonymous telephone callers.[1]

GAIT

Any identification based on recollection of physical characteristic of a person in question by friends and relatives is unreliable. The gait may be altered by an accident or by design. [1, 2, 3]

TRICKS OF MANNER AND HABIT

They are frequently hereditary, e.g. left handed-ness. Jerky movement of shoulder or face is an individual characteristic. [1-3, 5, 6]

MEMORY AND EDUCATION

They are sometimes useful, especially in cases of impostors. [1-3]

REFRENCE

1. MahantaPutul, Modern Textbook of Forensic Medicine And Toxicology *(2014)*,Jaypee Brothers Medical Publishers, Darya Ganj, New Delhi. 69-110

2. Parikh C.K., Parikh's textbook of medical jurisprudence forensic medicine and toxicology, *sixth edition (2011)*, C.B.S. Publishers and Distributors, Ansari Road, Darya Ganj, New Delhi, pg.no. 2.1- 2.38

3. Modi. Jaising. P, Textbook of Medical Jurisprudence And Toxicology, Twenty *First Edition (1997)*, N.M. Tripathi Private Limited, Bombay.pg.no. 18- 63

4. Forensic medicine, pg.no 20-40

5. A.K. Dutta, forensic medicine and toxicology, 4th edition (2006), current distributors, pg.no 10-31

6. C. k. Basu, Forensic medicine and toxicology, Reprint (2007),Current book distributor, pg.no.11-28

7. Usmani hammad,tib ul qanoon, universal publication house Allahabad, 1967 and 1976 pg.no.51-87

8. www.wikipedia.com

9. Krishan Vij Textbook of Forensic medicine and Toxicology, 4th Edt.

Chapter 3

MEDICOLEGAL AUTOPSY

Medicolegal autopsy

Autopsy [auto=self; opsi=view] literally means to see for oneself. A medicolegal autopsy [necropsy] or postmortem examination [necros–dead; opsi=view, post=after; mortem=death] is a special type of scientific examination of a body carried out under the laws of the state mainly for protection of its citizens and to assist the identification and prosecution of the guilty in cases of unnatural deaths. As such, it requires state permission and must meet with certain essential requirements. [1]

Medicolegal autopsy is the post-mortem examination of the dead body for the purpose of ascertaining the cause of suspicious or unnatural deaths, sent to doctors by police, Magistrates and courts law.

Besides medicolegal autopsy, dead bodies may be dissected for the purpose of acquiring knowledge on Human Anatomy and for confirmation of clinical diagnosis of cause of death and assessment of pathological changes in different organs [pathological autopsy].

For study of HUMAN ANATOMY, unclaimed dead bodies, duly embalmed, are dissected. Pathological autopsies are done after obtaining written consent from next of kin of the deceased. Pathological autopsies are essential not only for enriching medical science but also for better medical diagnosis and management for future patients.

To avoid cases under Consumer Protection Act [CPA] and Medical Negligence changer on Hospital deaths, the attending doctors should try to perform increasing number of Pathological autopsies. If an allegation of Medical negligence is made against the attending Doctor, Officer-in-Change in Local Police station is to arrange for medicolegal Postmortem examination to prove or disprove such changes against the attending Doctor. [2]

- **Forensic pathology** deals with the investigation of sudden, unexpected and/or violent deaths that includes determining the cause of death and the circumstances of how the death occurred.
- **Autopsy*** refers to the systematic examination of a dead person for medical, legal and/or scientific purpose.

It is of three types:
  i.   **Academic:** dissection carried by students of anatomy.

ii.   **Pathological, hospital or clinical:** Done by pathologists to diagnose the cause of death or to confirm a diagnose. Physician cannot order these autopsies without the consent signed by the next of kin.

iii. **Medico-legal:** types of scientific examination of a dead body carried out under the laws of the state for the protection of rights of citizens. The basic purpose of this autopsy is to establish the cause and manner of death. [3]

PURPOSE/OBJECTIVES

Who, when, where, why, how and what are the questions that the autopsy assists in answering. The objectives of medico-legal autopsy are: [3]

1. To determine the identity of the person.
2. To determine the cause of death, whether natural or unnatural;
a. If unnatural, whether suicide, homicide, or accident, and
b. in all cases but more important in homicide, to collect and document trace evidence, if any, left   by the accused on the victim.
c. To identify the weapon, person, or person responsible for death.
d. in case of fatal wounding, to determine the volitional activity possible after such trauma.
3. To estimate the approximate time since death [1]
4. In dead new born infants to determine the question of live-birth and viability i.e., whether dead born or still or died a natural or unnatural death after live-born [2]
5. In case of mutilated, fragmented or skeletal remains, to determine if they are human; and if human, the probable cause of death and approximate time since death , and
6. To restore the body to the best possible cosmetic appearance before it is released to the relatives. [1]

CODES [Prerequisites and protocols]

1. The medicolegal autopsy should be conducted in a place specially authorized and designed for the purpose [e.g. Mortuary] and by a Medical officer authorized by the Government. However, in exhumation it may be carried out in an open space close to the grave, but the place must be screened off. In such cases final autopsy mat be done in a Morgue.

2. Official requisition [inquest report] in duplicate authorizing the autopsy, from the Police, Magistrate or court must be obtained along with as dead body challan showing place and time of dispatch of the dead body by the officer making inquest.

3. The autopsy should be performed without undue delay. Even if the body id decomposed autopsy should be performed as certain important finding mat still be detected.

4. The medical Officer should be first read the inquest report carefully and find out the apparent cause of death mention from the appearance and surrounding of the body, and obtain all the available details of the case from the case sheet,

accident register, etc., so that attention may be directed to the salient points, while doing the postmortem examination. [2]

5.   Identification of dead body is very important. A Police Officer or any other authorized person and two relatives should identify the dead body, in front of the Autopsy Surgeon. The names of those who identify the body must be recorded. In unidentified bodies, the marks of identification, race, religion, sex, age, dental formula, photograph and fingerprints should be taken. [3]

6.   No unauthorized person should be present at the autopsy. The investigating Police Officer may however be present.

7. The examination should be conducted preferably in day light, because colour changes, such as jaundice, changes in bruises, changes in post-mortem staining etc., and may not be appreciated accurately in artificial light. If the body is received late in the evening a preliminary examination may not be done to note the external appearance, the body and rectal temperature and the appearance of the superficial injuries, extent of post-mortem lividity and rigor mortis etc. further post-mortem examination may be conducted on the next day, as early as possible.

8. While the autopsy is conducted – the findings of examination should be noted with sketches and photograph of the important injuries and findings.

9. All the body parts and every organ must be examined be dissecting them out from the cavities: thoracic, abdominal and cranial cavities[2]

10. Ordinarily, a dead body is sent to the morgue but in exceptional cases the medical officer mat be taken to the place where a dead body is lying. In that case he should note the place and nature of the soil where he found the dead body, and also its position especially as regards the hand and feet and the state of the clothes, if any.

11. He should also note, in the case of death from violence, the position of the body in reference to surrounding objects, such as sharp stones and the like, contact with which, it might be alleged, had produced the injury, also whether any blood stains where visible on such object or anywhere near the corpes, and whether any weapons were lying near it.

12.   The ground in the vicinity should be carefully searched for the presence of footprints and evidence of any struggle.

13. In case of suspected death from poisoning, he should note whether any appearance as of vomited matter, etc., was present in the neighborhood of the body. Much valuable evidence can be obtained be proper investigation at the sense of crime.

14. Whenever to persons or objects come in contact with each other they leave evidence of transference of material from each other in the form of finger prints, fibers, dust, hair, avulsed nails, etc. and provide irrefutable evidence for the scientific investigation at the very scene of crime.

15. Hence accurate sketch of the scene, photograph and selective collection of material and the initial recordings of the body temperature at regular intervals, extent of rigor mortis, hypostasis, presence of possible weapons, ligature, blood stains, evidence of struggle, medicine bottles, ova and maggots etc., collection of saliva or semen swabs by a forensic pathologist is of great help.

16. It is better to protect the different parts of body in plastic bags or pads to prevent loss of contact tracers, while it is being removed to a mortuary. [4]

MEDICOLEGAL AUTOPSY REPORTS

The medicolegal autopsy [Post-Mortem] report consists of the three parts, namely:

I. Introduction of preamble

This should state the authority [Police station case reference] ordering the examination, time of dispatch and arrival of the dead body at the mortuary, the date, time and place of examination the name, age and sex of the deceased, information furnished in the inquest report and the means by which dead body was identified.

II. Body of report i.e. facts observed on examination

This consist of Post-Mortem finding which comprise of complete description of the external and internal examination of the body with exact measurement and description of injuries, ligature mark etc. if necessary may be drawn on back page of P.M. report or on a separate sheet.

III. Conclusion or opinion

The conclusion or opinion regarding the cause of death and other point are based on the post-mortem findings.

The opinion should be to the point without any ambiguity. The opinion should be honest, objective and scientific. Autopsy surgeon should sign the report and state hid name in Block Letters and designation. Qualification or degrees may be mentioned after his name.

The Medicolegal Autopsy Reports [P.M.] prepared by the Medical Officer in triplicate by carbon process by own handwriting of the Autopsy surgeon ass per Police Regulation of West Bengal.

With the advent of computer the question of modernizing the writing P.M. report by the way computer printing of Post-Mortem findings and opinion etc. on the Model P.M. report from [video recorded P.M. examination for custodial death] in all P.M. examination, is being proposed be some Autopsy Surgeon, but it requires sanction from Home and Police Deptt. Of Govt. for a legal implementation of this proposal.

It is usually not admitted as documentary evidence unless the concerned doctor attends the court and testifies the facts under an oath. Defense Counsel can cross examine the doctor over the report. Occasionally Law courts accept the P.M. report as an exhibit due to nonavailability of Autopsy surgeon etc. [2]

PROCEDURE FOR MEDICOLEGAL AUTOPSY
INSTRUMENTS :
1. Scalpels of different sizes.
2. Organ knives of 6" and 10" blade.
3. Cartilage knives of 5 ¼" and 4" blade.
4. Brain knife 10" blade.
5. Resection knife.
6. Cotlin.
7. Bistoury – probe pointed.
8. Scissors –blunt and sharp -8", 6" and 11" for bowel.
9. Fine point Mayo scissors -5 ¼" also dissecting scissors -5" with one probe point for coronary arteries.
10. Bone cutter -10" straight and angled.
11. Rib shears -9 ½.
12. Dissecting forceps of different sizes, spencer-Wells forceps.
13. Barnard's saws 9" and 11"and an electric saw with accessories.
14. Lands hinged coronet.
15. Set of half curved and double curved needles.
16. Probe with eye
17. Chisels straight and spine with locating point.
18. Gourge – ¾" blade.
19. Hammer with wrench end.
20. Box wood mallet with metal bands.
21. A metal or plastic measuring tape.
22. Measuring and graduated glass containers.
23. China plates.
24. Basins to contain water.
25. A pair of thick India Rubber gloves with gauntlets or photographic gloves.
26. Sponges.
27. Machine for weighing organs.
28. At least two wide mouthed, white glass bottles [with glass stoppers] of about one liter capacity to contain portions of viscera.
29. Few glass slides and test tubes.
30. A hand lens, particularly useful for distinguishing apparently incised wounds from lacerated wounds on the scalp and over hard bones. Facilities for X-Ray and photographing are essential are often very useful. [4]

There are two types of examination:
1.   External examination.
2.   Internal examination.

EXTERNAL EXAMINATION

Those observations which pertain to the objectives of a medicolegal autopsy are specially looked for and these include:

I.   Data for identification.
II. Detailed examination of clothing and whole body pointing directly or indirectly to the cause of death.
III. Photograph or sketches of evidential value, and
IV. Data indicative of time since death. [1]

The following steps should be followed for the external examination:

1.   The body should be identify by the police constable and the chaukidar, who brought it to the mortuary. It should also be identified by a relative or friend of the deceased present on the spot. These persons will be required to give evidence in court of having identified the body in the presence of the medical officer holding the post-mortem examination in case a person is tired for having caused the death of the deceased.

2.   In the case of an unknown body, a general appearance of the body describing the race, sex, age, stature, features, scars, colour and distribution of hair on the body, tattoo-marks; teeth and occupational characteristics etc., should be noted for the purpose for identification. The body should be photographed and the fingers prints take.

The police should arrange for such a body to be photographed at once, before it gets decomposed. The photograph is worthless after the features have become bloated and distorted from putrefaction, but often bodies are photographed even after advanced putrefaction [4]

3.   The points relating to the probable cause of death must include everything that is indicative of the mode of death. In forensic work, the common causes of unnatural death are violence and poisoning.

4.   The clothes should be described as regards its natural and condition, noting any tears, loss of buttons, or disarrangement [indicating possible struggle]. Cuts, holes, burns, or blackening from firearm discharges should be described [1]

The clothes should be removed carefully without tearing them to avoid confusion with signs of struggle. If they cannot be removed intact they should be cut parrale to the stich lines [2]

Stains of blood, saliva, semen, vomit or faecal matter, pieces of glass, bits of paint, fibers, hair etc. should be described and preserved for chemical analysis.

5.   In case of a cord or ligament round the neck, its exact position, manner and application of a knot or knots and its material should be noted.

6.   Height, weight and general state of body built development and nourishment are noted [2]

Age should be given from the presence of the teeth and other appearances. If owing to rigor mortis, the jaw cannot be opened to count the teeth, the cheeks should be cut to expose them. [4]

7. Nail scrapping should be taken before the clothing's are removed. Any substance or matter [including fibers like hair] held or adherent in the hand should be removed with match stick and placed in envelopes. Ideally tem small envelopes are labeled, one for each finger, and each envelope, is sealed. [2]

8. Time since death should be noted from the rectal temperature of the body, post-mortem staining, rigor mortis, stage of putrefaction, ova of flies and maggots, and even from the degree of digestion of the stomach contents which, however, only yields evidence of doubtful value.

9. The condition of the body, whether stout, emaciated, or decomposed, should be mentioned.

The eyes should be examined for softening of the eyes ball and the opacity of the cornea and lens should be noted particularly in vehicular accidents. The state of the pupils, their colour, and any evidence of petechial hemorrhage or injury to periorbital tissue should be noted. [4]

10. The condition of natural orifices, viz, nose, mouth, ears, urethra, vagina, and anus, should be observed and any change from the normal noted. Irritants, e.g., cocaine, severely ulcerate nasal mucous membrane. Any smell, e.g., of alcohol, insecticides, etc., should not escape attention nor the presence of a foreign body. The mouth may reveal foreign bodies, drugs, damaged teeth, injured gums and lips [ruptured frenum of child abuse], and the bitten tongue of epilepsy. Any abnormal position of the tongue in relation to the teeth should be noted. The ears are examined for leakage of blood or CSF. Sample of discharge from urethra. Vagina and anus should be taken on swabs [or smears prepared on slides]. [1]

11. The hand should be examined for nay article, such as hair, fragments of clothing or a weapon grasped by them or the presence of mud or blood on them or under the nails. Scrapings from under the nails can easily be taken in an envelope by a pointed match stick or the point of a double folded filter paper and properly labeled. Dust in the cerumen is also helpful. [4]

12. Colour and condition of skin of face blue [cyanosis] with petechiae and congestion and the presence of stain on the skin from blood, mud, vomit, faeces, corrosive, or other poisons or gun-powder over the areas are noted in details.

The presence of edema of legs, surgical emphysema the chest are specially looked for etc.

13. Scalp is to examine for any foreign matter in the scalp hair should be removed with forceps and if necessary after combing them to obtain trace evidence. Sample of both cut and pulled hair from at least six labeled. Palpation of scalp for fracture, local swelling, trauma are to be made. [2]

14. After washing the body a careful search for the presence of injuries or marks of violence should be made all over the body from head to foot, on the front as

well as on the back. Any injection mark on the body should be carefully noted. In the case of a female body the hair of the head should be removed to examine the scalp. In ant injuries are found on the body, the should be photographed or marked carefully on sketches, before they are described in detail in the post-mortem report.

Such a procedure is very helpful in enabling the magistrate and counsel of both sides to understand the exact nature, extent and situation of the injuries on the body.

Bruises and abrasions, if any, should be described as regards their length, breadth, direction, colour and their exact position. Bruises should be incised to find out if they were inflicted before or after death and to differentiate them from suggilation.

Wounds due to assault, defense, accident etc. if present, should be described as regards their nature, dimensions, direction and position. The condition of their edges, presence of any coagulated blood between them, or evidence of bleeding into the wound nearby tissue should be mentioned. A hand lens may be used. The exact size ought to be noted with a measuring tape and some fixed bony points should be taken to describe their exact position. The means by which they were inflicted should also be noted.

Deep or penetrating wounds should not be investigated by means of a probe, until the body is opened.

In case of gunshot wound the course and direction of the bullet should be ascertained by dissection rather than by the use of probe, and the injured nerves and blood-vessels, if any are found, should be noted. If there is only one opening, a search should be made for the bullet, which must be preserved, it must not be washed but dried.it should be remembered that a bullet takes a very tortous and erratic course in its passage through the body and sometimes X-Ray are necessary for location a bullet. A note should be made, if the skin in the vicinity of the wound is blackened and if the hair is scorched.

Ligature marks, finger marks or abrasions, if present on the neck, should be noted.

In the case of burns, their position, external and degree should be mentioned, as also the manner of their causation as to whether they were caused by fire, scalding fluids, corrosive sor explosive. [4]

15. If a cardiac pacemaker is present, it should be removed lest the heating of the mercury batteries result in an explosion in the crematorium or cause environmental pollution, in due course, when buried. It is also necessary to check if the pace maker was still functioning properly [electrical performance] especially if death was sudden and apparently due to cardiac malfunction [as opposed to pneumonil!]. [1]

16. All the bones should be carefully examined for the presence of fracture and the joints for dislocations. If any fracture is present, the soft part overlying the

fractured piece should be dissected and examined for laceration or ecchymosis even though no abnormal mobility or crepitus is detected.

Lastly, all the external injuries should be compared with those noted in the descriptive roll supplied by the police and any discrepancy should be mentioned in the report. [4]

17. In the case of a body of a newly born infant where the question of live birth and viability is to be determined, it is necessary:
   a) To examine the umbilical cord
   b) To note the shape of the chest
   c) To look the certain ossific centers.

The umbilical cord is examined for its total length when possible, how it is severed, and the nature of any ligature thereon; and its condition, whether dry, healing, or separated. The chest is examined for its shape, whether arched or flat. The ossific centers in the following bones are looked for:
   1) Calcaneum [20th week]
   2) Talus [28th week]
   3) Lower end of femur [36the week]. [1]

INTERNAL EXAMINATION

It is convenient to start the examination with the cavity chiefly affected. All three major cavities of the body, i.e. skull, thorax and abdomen should be opened and examined as a routine. The choice as to which part of body is to be opened first – skull or the body cavities is left to the dissector.

   ➤ In suspected head injury, open the skull and then the thorax and the abdomen, but some authors are of the view that should be opened after blood has been drained out by opening the heart.
   ➤ In suspected asphyxial deaths due to compression of neck, open the skull and abdomen first followed by dissection of the neck. The draining out of blood from neck vessels via the skull provides a comparatively cleaner field for the study of neck structure.
   ➤ In all other cases, the thorax and abdomen are opened then the skull. [3]

Professor Harvey Little John recommends the examination of the head first in cases of alleged infanticide so that examined may have an opportunity of inspecting the contents of the skull before the blood can possibly drain away during examination of the thorax and trunk and also because he will be better able to interpret appearance in the lungs when they are examined.

Every organ contained in the cavities must always be examined, but the spinal cord need not ordinarily be examined unless there is suspicion of some injury to the vertebral column or the alleged cause of death is due to some sprinal poison or some such disease as tetanus. In that case it should be examined last of all. [4]

The spinal cord need not be examined except in cases of:
1) Local injury
2) Sudden death following trauma without apparent local injury
3) Death from convulsions
4) Battered babies
5) When such an examination is specially requested by the investigating officer.

If the naked eye examination fails to reveal the cause of death, the medical officer should take appropriate specimens for histology and culture. [1]

SKIN INCISIONS

Skin incisions are three types.
I.   **I-SHAPED INCISION:** extending from the chin straight down to the symphysis pubis and avoiding the umbilicus [because the dense fibrous tissue is difficult to penetrate with needle, when the body is stitched after autopsy]. Most common method followed.
II. **Y-SHAPED INCISION:** Straight line of Y corresponding to xiphisternum to pubis incision and forks of Y runs down below the breast and extending towards the acromion process. It is desirable in those cases [especially females] where it is customary to keep a dressed body foe viewing for sometimes after death.
III. **MODIFIED Y-SHAPED INCISION:** An incision is made in middle form suprasternal notch to symphysis pubis. The incision extends from suprasternal notch over the clavicle to its center on both sides and then passes upward over the neck behind the ears. It is used when a detailed study of neck organs is required, e.g. hanging or strangulation.

EVISCERATION METHODS

I.   **En masse:** This method, described by Letulle, involves removing most of the internal organs in one full swoop. It is rapid technique for removing the organs from the body although the ensuing dissection I the attachment intact.

II. **Virchow's method:** This method of evisceration is simply removal of individual organ one by one with subsequent dissection of that isolated organ. It is useful in assessing individual organ pathology, a quick an effective method, if the pathological interest is in a single organ.

III. **En bloc removal:** It is a compromise between the above methods and most widely used in UK. Ghon developed this method, which is relatively quick, but preserves most of the important inter-organ relationship.

IV. **In situ dissection:** This method developed by Rokitansky, is rarely performed which involves dissecting the organs in situ with little actual evisceration being performed prior to dissection. It may be the method of choice on patient with highly transmissible diseases.

No matter which dissection technique is utilized to eviscerate, the autopsy surgeon needs to perform a dissection specific to the organ in question.

- Hollow structures, such as blood vessels and GI tract [esophagus, stomach and intestine] is cut opened in order to reveal the pathology present inside.

- For solid organs, mat parallel cuts, in a fashion similar to slicing a loaf of bread is done.

  Whenever indicated, a small portion of each organ is preserved in formalin for histopathological examination. [3]

HEAD / SKULL

I. The body lies flat on its back with a wooden block underneath the shoulder and the head resting firmly on a head rest. The scalp is incised from mastoid to mastoid over the vertex taking care not the cut large masses of hair. This is done by the inserting the scalpel at the right mastoid with the cutting edge facing the dissector and cutting the full thickness of scalp from beneath outward over a coronal line curving over the vertex to the opposite mastoid.

The scalp flaps are reflected forward and backwards and note is made of any injury or oedema. Any depressed fracture, if present, is recorded with its dimensions and contour.

II. The temporalis muscle is incised about its middle on each side. The skull cap is swas and removed, the line of severance following a point just above the superciliary ridges in front and through the occiput behind, and preferably making an angle of 120 degrees between the anterior and posterior cuts.

This ensures that the skull cap will not shift on reconstruction of the body. The removal of the skull cap is facilitated by gently inserting and twisting a chisel at various places through the cut taking care not produce and post-mortem fracture or extend the existing ones, and to avoid any damage to the meninges and brain.

III. The dura is examined for the outside for extradural haemorrhage, and the superior sagittal sinus for antemortem thrombus. The weight and/or volume of extradural haemorrhage, if present, is recorded. An antemortem thrombus in the superior sagittal sinus can lead to back pressure in the bridging veins crossing the subdural space resulting in subdural haemorrhage. In old persons, the meninges over the vertex are often white and thickened with small calcified patches [arachnoid granulation].

IV. The dura is cut olong the line of severed skull cap and pulled gently from front to back while cutting the falx cerebri. A note is made of subdural and subarachnoid haemorrhage, if any. The weight and volume and volume of subdural haemorrhage, if present, is recorded, and its effect on the brain-flattening, asymmetry, etc., assessed.

V. If the injury is recent [hours] and blood is not preserved at or near the time of injury, the extradural and subdural haematoma can be preserved for toxicological analysis, especially alcohol and drugs.

VI. Four findings for left hand are inserted between the frontal lobes and skull and the frontal lobes drawn backward. The nerves and vessels as they emerge from skull are cut with right hand, A CSF sample is obtained by aspiration with a Pasteur pipette from the base. The tentorium is cut along the superior border of the petrous bone. The cervical cord, first cervical nerves, and vertebral arteries, are cut as far below as possible, and the brain along with cerebellum removed.

During the procedure, the brain is supported throughout with left hand. It is weighed and transferred to a clean dish for subsequent examination.

VII. The remaining venous sinuses are examined for antemortem thrombi.

VIII. The pituitary is removed by chiselling away the posterior chinoid processes and incising the diaphragm of sella turcica around its periphery. Incing the diaphragm alone is sufficient in many cases. The gland is examined, if necessary, after fixation in 10% formal saline, for tumor, infarct, atrophy, or any other pathological condition.

IX. The dura is pulled out to examine the base of skull and the rest of cranial cavity for ant fracture. If this is not done, even a big fracture mat be overlooked.

X. wedge shape portion of petrous temporal bone is removed to examine the mastoid for ant collection of pus, haemorrhage, or fluid in the middle ear [some drowning victims show haemorrhage in the middle and inner ear]. The orbits and air victims show haemorrhage if necessary.

XI. The skull cap is inspected for fracture by holding it against light or tapping it to elicit a cracked sound.

XII. The brain is examined for any swelling, shrinkage, or herniation; it's upper and lateral surfaces for asymmetry or flatting of convolutions; circle of willis for aneurysm; and smaller cerebral arteries for embolism.

XIII. The cerebellum is separated at the pons transversely just below the cerebral peduncles.

XIV. The brain is cut in serial coronal sections about 1 cm apart [or cut obliquely at intracerebral fissure] exposing the basal ganglia, lateral ventricles and white matter. It is examined for thickness of grey matter, haemorrhage or other abnormality. Shrinkage of cerebral cortex [grey matter] is common in chronic alcoholic, cerebral fat emboli which have completely obstructed the small vessels of brain may be visible or naked eye as punctate haemorrhage in the white matter. Petechial haemorrhage

I white matter are commonly found in death from anaphylactic shock. In head injury, oedema seems in white matter around or deep to contusions, lacerations, or ischaemic lesions. If there are wounds of the brain, successive sections parallel to the wounded surfaces are made till the whole depth of the wound is revealed.

XV.   The cerebellum is cut vertically through the vermis to expose the fourth ventricle. An oblique cut is made through each hemisphere to expose the dentate nucleus. Any disease, injury, or haemorrhage, if present, is noted.

SPINAL CORD

Either an anterior or posterior approach can be used. The examination of thoracic spinal column is facilitated by the anterior approach. High cervical injuries are best demonstrated by the posterior approach, which is in common use.

I.   The body is turned over on to the face with a block beneath the thorax. A routine midline incision is made from the base of skull to sacrum. The paraspinal muscles and fasciae are scraped off from the spinous processes and laminae. A laminectomy is performed on each vertebra by sawing through the entire lenghth of spine on each side of the spinous processes. The laminae of first cervical vertebra are not severed or else the head will move too freely on the spine. The spinous processes and attached laminae are removed en masse. The spinal cord can also be removed from the front after the trunk is eviscerated

II.   The dura is examined for any pathological condition, such as inflammation, haemorrhage, suppuration, or tumour. It is cut in midline. The spinal nerves are cut from below upwards as they pass through the spinal foramina. The cord is separated at the foramen magnum, carefully lifted from the vertebral column, and placed on the table.

III.   After some fixation usually of several days duration, the cord is cut transversely at several places and examined for ant pathological condition such as softening, crushing, haemorrhage, infarction, inflammation, or intramedullary tumour, and some tissue is retained for histological examination.

IV.   The vertebral column is examined for fracture [especially of the odontoid process and cervical vertebrae], disc protrusion, tumour, dislocation, and vertebral collapse.

Bruising under the paravertebral fascia should be taken as indication of whiplash injury of fractured of the cervical vertebrae which should be specially looked for. [1]

THORAX

Before examining the thorax, both the cavities, the thorax and the abdomen should be opened by making a longitudinal incision from above the middle of the sternum to the pubic bone, keeping wide away from any wounds existing in its line. In infant bodies the incision should be carried a little to the of the umbilicus.

The integument, fascia and muscles should now be reflected and examined for extravasation of the blood in their inner surface. The abdominal cavity should be examined before the chest cavity is opened. The colour and appearance of the abdominal viscera, as also the position of the diaphragm with respect to the ribs [especially in full term newly –born infant bodies] should be noted. It should also be noted if there is any collection of blood, serum, pus or faecal matter in the cavity.

• After this preliminary, the examination of the thorax should be proceed with. The ribs and sternum should first be examined for evidence of fracture and then the cavity of thorax should be opened by dividing the ribs at their cartilages and the sternum at the sternoclavicular junctions with the costatome and lifting up the sternum separating it from the underlying parts without injuring them [4]

LUNGS:-

I. The plural cavities should be examined for the presence of adhesions, foreign bodies, pleuritis, petechial haemorrhage, injury, effusion, hemothorax, pneumothorax, pyothorax is noted.

II. Normal lungs weigh 250-400g each in an adult, but may weigh >1kg in case of severe cardiac failure or diffuse alveolar damage.

III. It is conventional to cut open from large to small airways, from medial to lateral to include all lobes are segments opening along the branches as they are encountered. Impression of the parenchymal appearance and texture is noted and apical disease like old tuberculous cavities or fungal balls can also be demonstrated.

IV. The parenchyma is squeezed and any pus or fluid expressed in noted. 3

V. The lungs should be removed from the cavity. After noting the condition of the lungs regards oedema, emphysema, elasticity, atelectasis etc., they should be cut open for evidence of disease, congestion, injury, Tardieu's spot, etc., and the bronchi should be examined for the presence of pent up expectoration, pus or any foreign body. 4

VI. After the horizontal slicing through each lobe with a brain-knife is made to inspect the rest of the parenchyma.

VII. It is occasionally preferable to make large horizontal slices through the whole lung rather than opening the airway and vessels in cases or large lesion [e.g. Carcinoma].

Dissection of the vessels:-

• The cause of pulmonary veins into the lung is traced and thrombosis and atheroma is looked for, the latter being associated with pulmonary hypertension. An antemortem embolus may be coiled and when the straightened resembles a castoff the vessel from which the thrombus originated, usually in the leg. Massive pulmonary emboli may block either the main trunk of the pulmonary artery or one of the major pulmonary vessels, more commonly on the right side.

I. Antemortem thrombus is weakly adherent to the lining endothelium, with a pale, granular and transversely ridged surface because of alternating layers of platelets and fibrin.

II. Postmortem thrombus is weakly adherent to the lining endothelium, dark-red, glistening and febrile. It is of two types:

    a. Black current-jelly: when blood clots rapidly, a soft, lumpy, uniformly dark-red, rubbery and moist clot is produced.

    b. Chicken-fat: when red cells sediment before blood coagulates, the red cells produce a clot similar to the first, but above this a pale or bright –yellow layer of serum and fibrin is seen.[3]

HEART :-

I. The heart is held at the apex, lifted upwards and separated from other thoracic organs by cutting the inferior and superior vena cava, pulmonary vessels, and ascending aorta as far away as possible from the base of the heart.

II. The size and weight of the heart is noted. Adult heart weighs about 250-300 g. Hearts the weigh too much are at risk for sudden, lethal arrhythmias.

III. Many approaches method can be taken to dissect the heart. The appropriate method is selected on the basis of the age of the patient and any suspected abnormality.

IV. The overall anatomy of the heart needs to be evaluated for any congenital anomalies. The condition of the valves, presence and degree of atheroma in the valves and the intima of the large vessels is noted. Any ischemic lesion is searched for. The state of the mayocardium, size of the chamber, thickness of right and left ventricle, state of endocardium [subendocardial haemorrhage in the left ventricle], valvular lesions, and condition of the aorta with regards to any aneurysm, atherosclerosis, or syphilitic aortitis [tree bark appearance] is noted.

Examination of the heart:

Coronary artery disease is seen more commonly than valvular heart disease. The myocardium is examined for fibrosis or recent infarct. The myocardium infarct is easily identifiable when it is of more than 12 h of age. If an infarct is identified, sections from its central and peripheral zones are useful in dating the onset of ischemic damage and determining any recent extension.

Examination of coronary arteries [in situ examination]:

The extramural coronary arteries are examined by making a serial cross-sectional incision about 3-5 mm apart, in order to evaluate for atherosclerotic narrowing, the most common site being 1cm away from the origin of the left coronary artery.

The narrowest segments and any areas containing thrombi should be selected for microscopic examination.

The anterior descending branch of the left coronary artery is cut downwards along the front of the septum, then the circumflex branch on the opposite side of the mitral valve. The presence of acute coronary lesions, viz. plaque rupture, plaque haemorrhage or thrombus is noted. The extent of coronary artery atherosclerosis is categorized based by the plaque. Anything <50% is considered mild, while 50-75% is considered moderate and > 75% is severe.

I.   Another method to examine the heart is the inflow-outflow method or following the direction of blood flow. First, the right atrium is opened, followed by the tricuspid valve, and then the pulmonic valve. Next, the left atrium is opened, followed by the mitral valve and the aortic valve. During opening, the valve should be examined before being cut and valve orifice measured, special section can be taken at this point to evaluate the conduction [electrical] system of the heart.

II.   Another lesser used method is the short axis or ventricular slicing method. With the heart in the anatomical position, the first slice is made through the heart at a point about 3 cm from the apex separating it from the remainder of the heart.

Further complete slices are then made in parallel to this slice, 1cm apart , until reaching below the antrioventricular valves. The remainder is then examined by opening along the path of blood flow. It is useful if ischemic myocardial disease is suspected as it clearly demonstrates the distribution of infraction. Examination of coronary arteries should precede then examination of heart.

- **Examination of valve:** The circumference of the valve is measured. The circumereance of mitral valve is 8-10.5cm [mean 10cm] and admits two fingers; tricuspid valce is 10-12.5 cm [12cm] and admits three fingers; arotic valve is 6-8 cm [7.5cm] and pulmonary valve is 7-9 cm [8.5cm]. The decrease in circumference is suggestive of stenosis whereas increased circumference could be due to regurgitation or incomplete valves.

- **Ventricular hypertrophy:** An estimate is made by measuring the thickness of the ventricular walls at a point about 1 cm below the atrioventricular valve. The upper limits of normal are: left ventricle: 1.5 cm, right ventricle: 0.5 cm and atrial muscle: 0.2 cm.

SUBENDOCARDIAL HAEMORRHAGE

These are flame-shaped, confluent haemorrhages, and tend to occur in one continuous sheet rather than in patches, seen in the left ventricle, on the left side of the interventricular septum and on the opposing papillary muscles and adjacent columnae carnea.

Subendocardial haemorrhage is seen in:

- Severe loss of blood or shock
- Intracranial damage, such as head injury, cerebral edema, surgical craniotomy or tumours
- Death due to ectopic pregnancy, ruptured uterus, abortion, antepartum or postpartum haemorrhage
- Poisoning, e.g. arsenic or oleander.

AGONAL THROMBI: In case of a person dying slowly due to circulatory failure, a firm, stringy, tough, pale-yellow thrombus forms in the cavities, usually on the right side of the heart.

The pericardium is examined for presence of any pathology or injury. The content of the pericardium sac and its quantity is noted.

Pericardial effusion, cardiac temponade, subpericardial haemorrhage and constrictive pericarditis are looked for.

NECK

The neck structures are examined before removal of the thoracic organs so that the tongue, larynx, trachea and esophagus can be taken out along with the lungs. This helps in examination of the whole of the upper respiratory tract in its continuity.

In case of death due to alleged constriction of the neck, there may be fracture of hoyoid bone or thyroid cartilage with extravasation of the blood into the tissues and injury to carotid arteries, sternomastoid muscles or platysma. Compression of the neck with hard materials may cause injury to the cervical vertebrae and the corresponding part of the spinal cord. The level and extent of the other mechanical injuries on the neck are cautiously examined to know the type of injury and organs or structures injured resulting in death. 3

ABDOMEN

The recti muscles of abdomen are divided about 5cm above symphysis. A small slit is at first made big enough to admit the index and middle finger, and while the fingers are used to guard the underlying structure, knife is moved thus exposing the area from xiphisternum to pubis.

I. Thickness of fat in the wall is noted, condition of the peritoneal cavity and organs are first observed before the organs are disturbed. Presence or absence of any blood, pus or fluid, foreign body [bullet, etc.] in the cavity, or perforation or damage to any organ are especially looking for.

II. Amount of fat in the mesentery and omentum. The abnormalities and position of abdominal organs are described.

III. All the internal organs are examined in situ, including the diaphragm and then all the abdominal organs are taken out either enmasse with thoracic organs or they are individually taken out. 2

IV.   The peritoneum should be first examined for evidences of anhesions, congestion, inflammation, or exudation of lymph or pus. The abdominal and pelvic cavities should then be examined for presence of a serous, bloody, purulent fluid, or gastric contents. Now the abdominal organs should be removed and examined separately as below :-

STOMACH:

In ordinary circumstances the stomach is examined by making a cut while in situ for the contents as regards their quantity and quality and the degree of their digestibility. But in suspected poisoning the stomach should be remove after tying a double ligature 1" to 2" above the cardiac end and at the pyloric end. It should then be opened along the greater or lesser curvature in a thoroughly clean plate; after emptying the contents in a special glass bottle for being sent to the chemical examiner, its mucous surface should be carefully examined noting its appearance, and any suspicious particles found adherent thereto should be picked off with a pair of fareceps and placed in a separate small phial for chemical analysis.

The contents of the stomach should also be examined as regards their smell, colour and character and for the presence of any foreign particles or lumps; these, if present, should be felt between the thumb and index finger as to their roughness or smoothness.[4]

INTESTINE:

Small and large intestines are examined. Two ligatures are applied near duodenojejunal flexure and cut between them. The whole of small intestines is taken out of the body by cutting the attachments of mesentery to the jejunum ileum. The ascending colon is separated from the retroperitoneal tissues by incising the peritoneum along its right border. The peritoneum along its left border. The transverse and pelvic colons are taken out like the small intestine as they have mesocolons. Two ligatures are applied over the rectum and it is cut between them, and the whole bowel is thus removed.

The small intestine is opened along the line of mesenteric attachment and the large intestine along the anterior tenia. They are examined for congestion, inflammation, erosions, ulcers, perforation, bullets. The contents are also examined and first fifty centimetre of it is preserved for chemical analysis.[2]

LIVER:

The surface of the liver should be examined as regards its smoothness or roughness. If there is any injury to the injury to the liver, its nature and dimensions should be noted as well as the size and weight of the liver.

Normally the liver measures 12"× 7"× 3 ½". The organ should be cut open by deep incision in several places, and the colour, consistence and blood supply of its tissue should be carefully marked; at the same time the presence of an abscess, new growth or amyloid degeneration should be observed for.

The gall bladder should be opened and the presence or absence of bile stones and the character and quantity of the bile should be noted. The portal vein and hepatic artery should be explored.[4]

PANCREAS:

The pancreas is removed along with the stomach and duodenum. It is sliced by multiple sections at right angles to the long axis to expose the ductal system.[3] And it should also be examined and looked for fat necrosis.[4]

SPLEEN:

The spleen is removed by cutting through its pedicle; its size, weight, consistency, condition of capsule, rupture, injuries or disease is noted. Hilum should be inspected for splenunculi before dissecting the spleen.

 I.   Weight of normal spleen range from 130-170 g.

 II.   It is sectioned in its long axis, and the character of parenchyma, follicles and septa is noted.

 III. Inn case of septicaemia, the spleen will often be soft and liquefied and slicing may be impossible.

 IV.   With normal spleen or with amyloid deposition or portal hypertension slicing will be easy.[3]

KIDNEYS:

The kidney are removed after of the suprarenals, first left and then right, by incising the peritoneal fat just outside their lateral margins. They are measured and weighed. The kidney is held firmly between the thumb and fingers or between layers of gauze or sponge to prevent it from slipping. It is then cut horizontally through the convex border to the hilum and opened like two halves of a book. The capsule strips with difficulty in chronic nephritis, hypertensive nephrosclerosis, and pyelonephritis.

In these conditions, the kidneys are small in size and the cut surface appears granular. The cut surface is examined for the width of the cortex [about 1cm in a healthy subject], granularity of the surface, clarity of the corticomeduallary junctions, size of the renal pelvis, and any pathological process such as inflammation and degenerative changes. The renal pelvis is examined for calculi and evidence of inflammation.

A block is taken from the kidney in such a way as to include the mucosa of the renal pelvic and all other layers.[1]

BLADDER:

The bladder should be examined for congestion, haemorrhage, inflammation and ulceration of its mucous membrane, it may be opened in situ and its contents noted, but in a suspected case of poisoning the urine should be removed by catheter and preserved for chemical analysis, as it may sometimes give a valuable clue as to the nature of the poison.[4]

PROSTATE:

When the injured bladder is drawn backwards from symphysis pubis, the prostate is palpated, urethra divided distal to it, and prostate removed along with the urinary bladder. The prostate is then examined for enlargement or malignancy. Vertical sections are made through lateral and median lobes.

TESTES:

The deep aspects of the inguinal canal from beneath the reflected skin are cut. Spermatic cords are identified at the inguinal ring the testes are removed from the scrotum by separating them from the inside of scrotal sac by gentle blunt dissection. The testes and epididymis are cut longitudinally are examined for evidence of any disease or injury especially ecchymosis. Local bruising can be demonstrated in the tunica albuginea or the body of testis.

FEMALE GENITALIA:

In the case of abortion death, the entire genital tract is removed in one block as follows and then examined.

The legs are widely abducted, and an incision made outside the labia up to the symphysis pubis above and including the anus below. Another incision is made round the level of the pelvic brim and continued downwards to the pelvic outlet till it reaches the vaginal incision. The entire genital tract together with urinary bladder and rectum can then be removed. In other cases, the ovaries and fallopian tubes are freed from pelvic, the vagina cut at the upper third, and the whole block removed from the pelvic. Each organ e.g. ovary, fallopian tubes, and uterus, is separated. The uterus is then examined for its size, shape, weight and any abnormality. It is cut longitudinally to expose the endometrium, thickness of the uterine walls, and contents, if any – fluid, foreign body, or foetus. If a foetus is present, its intrauterine age is assessed. The ovaries are cut longitudinally and examined for corpora lutea. The fallopian tubes are cut across at intervals to examine patency.

The vagina is examined for marks of injury, presence of foreign body, condition of its mucous membrane, presence of rugae, and the condition and type of hymen.

Any fluid, if present, in the vaginal canal is aspirated for determination of acid phosphatase or creatine phosphokinase, blood group substances, and spermatozoa. The condition of the cervix and any marks of instrument injury are noted.

If any foreign body is found in the genital tract, it is preserved along with such portion or whole of the genital tract as deemed necessary.[1]

DISSECTION OF LIMBS:

Limb vessels are examined; bones are examined for fracture. Intact femur is preserved and marrow from femur is taken out in DNA laboratory after cutting a window over cortex for DNA studies.

After completing the autopsy, organs are replaced into the cavities and the dissected flaps are brought close together and wall is sutured. The body is handed over to the police constable accompanying it for disposal by the relatives. [2]

DESCRIPTION OF AN ORGAN

I.   **Size:** Measuring tape is used. A tense capsule indicated enlargement and loose capsule shrinkage.

II. **Shape:** Not any deviation from normal.

III. **Surface:** Most organs have dedicate, smooth, glistening and transplant capsule of serosa. Any thickening, roughening, dullness or opacity is noted.

IV. **Consistency:** The softness and firmness is appreciated by application of finger pressure.

V.   **Cohesion:** It is strength within the tissue that holds an organ together. It is judged by the resistance of the cut surface to tearing, pressure or pulling.

VI. **Cut surface:** Note colour and structural details.

After completion of autopsy, bloods fluid etc. are removed from the body cavities. The organs are replaced in the body and any excess space is packed with cotton or cloth, especially in the pelvis and the throat, where blood tends to leak. The dissected flaps are brought close together and sutured by using thin twine and large curved needle. The skull should be filled with remaining portion of the brain along with cotton or other absorbent material and the skull cap fitted in place.

The scalp is pulled back over the vault and the scalp stitched with thin strong twine. The body is washed with water, dried and covered with clothes and then handed over to the police constable accompanying it. [3]

LOBORATORY PROCEDURES

I.   Histology: From various internal organs, thin slices of tissues 0.5" cube size are removed and preserved in 10% formalin or 95% alcohol to prepare histological slides after tissue processing.

II. Microscopic examination of vaginal and anal swabs, urethral discharge, faeces and urine.

III. Blood and cerebro-spinal fluid are collected for biochemical examination. [2]

REPORT

After completing the post-mortem examination, a complete but concise report should be written in duplicate/triplicate using carbon papers. One copy is given to the investigating officer and another copy is retained for future reference [sometimes a third copy is made for hospital purpose or for the chemical examiner]. The report should a list specimens and samples retained for further examination.

- The report should be given on the day, as the details cannot be accurately recorded from memory, if there is too much of delay.

- If laboratory test have to be carried out, a provisional report is given and later after obtaining the reports, a supplementary report is given. In suspected cases of poisoning, the opinion should be kept reserved until the Chemical Examiner's report is received. In such cases, viscera should be preserved and histological and bacteriological examination may carry out. The conclusion that death was caused, toxicological, circumstantial and/or autopsy evidence.

- A definite opinion should be given whenever possible, but if the cause of death cannot be ascertained, it should be mentioned I the report. While giving cause of death, the word 'probably' should be avoided. It must be recognized that the determination of cause and manner of death are opinions, not facts. **The opinion of one autopsy surgeon can differ from another's.**

- If the cause of death is not found on autopsy, the opinion as to the cause of death should be given as 'undetermined', and the manner of death as 'unknown'.

DEMONSTRATION OF PNEUMOTHORAX

Pneumothorax occurs when a leakage through the pleura allows air to enter the plural cavity and the communication rapidly closes. It can be demonstrated by three ways during autopsy:

I.   The skin and subcutaneous tissue are reflected from the chest wall till the mid-axillary line, being careful not to open the plural cavity. Acre should be taken not to puncture the intercostal soft tissue and penetrate the plural space, as this releases air from an underlying pneumothorax. Water is poured into the angle between subcutaneous tissue and the chest wall, and the intercostal tissues below the water line are pierced with a blade. If pneumothorax is present, bubbles of air will be seen rising through the water.

II. Another method is possible before any incision is made. This involves introducing a wide bore needle attached to a 50ml syringe into the subcutaneous tissue over an intercostal space into the plural space. The plunger should be removed previously and the syringe filled with water. The water is observed for the presence of any bubbles. A similar procedure is then followed on the other side.

III. A third method involves post-mortem chest X-Ray and assessment in a manner similar to detection of a pneumothorax in the living patient.

DEMONSTRATION OF AIR EMBOLUS

For venous air embolus, a plane chest X-Ray before evisceration to demonstrate the pathology may be done. Examination of the retina should be performed with an ophthalmoscope for intravascular bubbles.

During dissection of the neck, the large neck veins should be carefully exposed, but not opened before the heart is dissected in situ, to avoid the confusion of air introduction during evisceration.

The abdomen is opened in the usual manner and the contents are moved to inspect the inferior vena cava for bubbles in the lumen through its transparent wall. There are three methods to demonstrate venous air embolus:

I.   The sternum is removed by dividing the ribs, being careful not to puncture the pericardial sac, and cutting through the sternum distal to the sternoclavicular joint.

The internal mammary vessels should be clamped. The anterior pericardial sac is opened and the external epicardial veins inspected for evidence of intraluminal bubbles. Water is introduced to fill the pericardial space. Once completely covered in water, the right atrium and ventricle are incised and careful inspection is made to identify any air bubbles which may escape.

II. Another method is by inserting a water-filled syringe [minus plunger] connected to a needle into the right ventricle, the syringe chamber observed for the presence of bubbles.

III. Pyrogallol test: A 2% pyrogallol solution mixed with sodium hydroxide is taken in a syringe. Gas is then aspirated for the right side of the heart and then shaken. The mixture will turn brown, if air is present. In the absence of air, the solution stays clear [indicating gas production by bacteria].

Arterial air emboli are unusual and usually result from traumatic injury involving the pulmonary veins or following introduction of air during cardiopulmonary bypass. Smaller volume of air is associated with such emboli and as such more difficult to demonstrate.

Systemic emboli may be verified by inspecting the intracranial vessels of the meninges and circle of Willis and then examining underwater after clamping the internal carotid and basilar arteries.[3]

DISPOSAL

Organs not required are replaced into the body cavities. The body is stitched, washed, and restored to the best possible cosmetic appearance, and handed over to the police, under a receipt, for further disposal.

PRESERVE, PACK AND LABEL

I.   Specimens for toxicological analysis and histological examination where necessary.

II.   Blood from leg [femoral vein] or arm [subclavian vein] for grouping, alcohol estimation, and toxicological analysis.

III.   Any tissue providing material evidence. Commonly, in most cases, blood, bile, urine, vitreous, and stomach contents provide the necessary info.[1]

PRESERVATION OF VISCERA

Viscera should be preserved in case of:

- Suspected death due to poisoning
- Deceased was intoxicated or used to drugs
- Cause of death could not be found after autopsy
- Accidental death involving driver of a vehicle or machine operator
- Death due to burns [if needed]
- Advanced decomposition
- Any case, if requested by the magistrate.[3]

If the patient is alive the following material should be preserved, preferably in the quantity mentioned:[1]

Material	Quantity
Vomit	300 ml [whole, if quantity is less]
Stomach washout	500 ml [whole, if quantity is less]
Blood	10 ml, preferably more, 100 ml
Urine	100-200 ml [whole, if quantity is less]

Viscera preserved during autopsy [routine]

S.NO.	Material	Quantity
1.	Stomach and its content	Whole
2.	Upper part of small intestine and its content	About 15-30 cm length [some say 100 cm]
3.	Liver [along with gallbladder]	300-500 g
4.	Kidney	Longitudinal half of each kidney
5.	Spleen	Whole
6.	Blood	10 ml
7.	Urine	100 ml

Additional viscera and material may be required in the following circumstances.

S.NO	Nature of poison	Material to be preserved.
1.	Alcohol	About 10ml blood from a peripheral vein and as much vitreous as can be withdrawn.
2.	Barbiturates	10ml blood.
3.	Carbon monoxide	About 10 ml blood.
4.	Chloroform	About 10 ml blood.
5.	Corrosive poison	Skin atleast 2.5 cm square from the affected ares and similar portion from the opposite are as control.
6.	Heavy metals [chronic poisoning by arsenic, anti – mony, etc.]	About 10 cm of shaft of long bone, about 5 g of plucked scalp hair, all finger or toe nails, skin of back, and a wedge of quadriceps muscles before opening the abdomen to avoid contamination.
7.	Hydrocyanic acid and cyanides	About 20 ml blood.
8.	Inhalation, or solvent and volatile substance	Tie off trachea. Collect entire lung and place in air tight container.
9.	Injected poison	Skin, subcutaneous tissue and muscle forming the injection track, and similar material from opposite side as control.
10.	Nux vomica and strychnine	Spinal cord, heart, and one half of brain.
11.	Opium	10 ml blood, gall bladder and its contents.
12.	Pesticides	Fatty tissue from abdominal wall or perinephric region and myoneural junction if possible.

S.NO	Special circumstances	Material to be preserved
1.	Criminal abortion	Vaginal, uterus, fallopian tubes, ovaries, urinary bladder, rectum, and abortion stick or foreign body in the genital track.
2.	Decomposed bodies	Insect eggs, maggots, and pupa.
3.	Embalmed bodies	Embalming fluid, bone marrow

4.	Exhumed bodies	Soil samples from above, beneath, and sides of the coffin, and control samples from distance away from the coffin. Any fluid found in the coffin.
5.	Extensive trauma in drunken individuals	Vitreous fluid for estimation of alcohol.
6.	Firearm injuries	Skin around the entrance and exit wounds
7.	Hydrophobia [rabies]	Brain for negri bodies [for pathologist]
8.	Stained clothes	Stained as well as surrounding unstained portion as control

COLLECTION OF SAMPLES

I. **BLOOD :** The cellular barrier of mucous and serous membrane breaks down after death, due to which substances [e.g. alcohol and barbiturates] in the stomach and intestine can migrate to the organs in the thorax and abdomen leading to erroneous results. Before autopsy, 10-20 ml of blood can be drawn from the femoral [best sample], jugular or subclvian vein by a syringe. Blood should never be collected from the plural or the abdominal cavities, as it can be contaminated with gastric or intestinal contents, lymph, mucus, urine, pus or serous fluid.

II. **CFS:** It is collected by lumber puncture or from the cisterna magna by inserting a long needle between the atlanto-occipital membranes. Direct aspiration of CFS can be done from the lateral ventricles or third ventricles after removal of the brain.

III. **VITREOUS HUMOR :** A fine hypodermic needle [20 gauge] attached to a syringe is inserted through the outer canthus into the posterior chamber of the eye, after pulling the eyelid aside, followed by aspiration of 1-2 ml of crystal clear is re-introduced through the needle to restore the tension in the globe for cosmetic reasons.

IV. **LUNGS:** In solvent abuse ['glue sniffing'] and death from gaseous or volatile substances, the lung is mobilized and the main bronchus tied off tightly with a ligature. The hilum is then divided and the bag is then sealed. Plastic [polythene] bags are not suitable, as they are permeable to volatile substances.

V. **URINE:** It can be collected in a suitable sterile or non-sterile 'universal container' for either microbiological or toxicological analysis by suprapibic puncture or when the bladder is opened. Before dissection, urine can be collected via catheter or abdominal wall puncture.

VI. **BONE:** About 200g is collected. It is convenient to remove about 10-15cm of the shaft of the femur. 3

VII.   **BONE MARROW:** The required quantity is obtained from sternum, femur, or vertebrae. 1

VIII.   **HAIR:** An adequate sample of head and pubic hair should be removed by plucking along with roots, and not by cutting, and preserved in separate containers [0.5g for DNA analysis, up to 10g for analysis of heavy metals].

IX.   **MAGGOTS:** These are dropped alive into boiling absolute alcohol or 10% hot formalin which kills them in an extended condition [to disclose the internal structure of the larvae]. If time of death is an issue, some larvae/maggots should be preserved alive for examination by an entomologist. Maggots may reveal the presence of drugs/poisons in decomposed bodies.

X.   **NAILS:** All the nails [fingers and/or toes] should be removed in their entirety and collected in separate envelopes.

XI.   **SKIN:** If there is needle puncture, the whole needle track and surrounding tissue should be excised. Control specimens should be taken from some other area on the opposite side of the body and preserved in a separate container. In firearm cases, a 2.5 cm square portion of skin around the entrance and exit wounds should be preserved.

- **Fibroblasts for tissue culture:** karyotype, metabolic assays, enzyme assays and diagnostic ultra structural studies can be performed on cultured fibroblasts. Skin, fascia, lung, diaphragm, muscle and cartilage are useful for fibroblast cell cultures.

- **Tissue for metabolic studies and nucleic acid analysis:** Liver, kidney, cardiac and skeletal muscle, and peripheral nerve obtained at autopsy may be used for biochemical studies in the diagnosis of inborn errors of metabolism. The tissue should be frozen rapidly in liquid nitrogen or dry ice and stored at -70degree.[3]

PRESERVATION OF SAMPLE

- The ideal sample are the once in which on preservation has been added and sent to CFSL within few hours. But, practically, it usually gets delayed.

- Few specimens are preserved at 4 degree until they are analysed. For long-term stronge, it has to be kept in freezer.

- In order that putrefaction mat not sent in and render chemical analysis difficult, certain preservatives are used.

1. **VISCERA**

   - The most common used preservation for viscera is saturated solution of common salt. It is easily available, cheap and effective preservative.

- In cases of suspected alkali or acid poisoning [except carbolic acid], rectified spirit is used. It is not used in cases of suspected poisoning with:

2. **Blood for toxicological analysis** [for alcohol, cocaine, cyanide and carbon monoxide (CO)] is preserved in sodium or potassium fluoride at the concentration of 10 mg/ml of blood and anticoagulant potassium oxalate, 30 mg/10 ml of blood.

   - Post-mortem samples are liable to production of concentrations of sodium fluoride are required to inhibit this.

   - Heparin and EDTA should not be used as anticoagulants, since they interfere with detection of methanol.

   - If blood is required only for grouping, no preservative is necessary and small amount of blood is well preserved by soaking in a blotter.

   - In case of suspected CO poisoning, a layer of 1-2 cm of liquid paraffin is needed immediately over the blood sample to avoid exposure to atmospheric oxygen.

   - If solvent abuse and anaesthetic death is suspected, the glass container should have a foil-lined lid to prevent gas from escaping [as gas can permeate rubber] and the container is completely filled to prevent gas from escaping in 'dead' air space.

   - Blood from haematological examination including glycosylated haemoglobin in diabetics should be sent in a clear glass container with anticoagulant [e.g. EDTA].

3. Urine is preserved by adding small amount of phenyl mercuric nitrate or thymol. Fluoride should be added to urine if alcohol, cyanide or cocaine is suspected in the sample.

4. Vitreous humour is preserved using sodium fluoride [10 mg/ml].

5. For bones, hair and nails preservative is not required. It has to be dried in normal temperature and sealed in plastic bag. But, bone marrow is preserved in a test tube containing 4-5 ml of 5% albumin-normal saline solution and stored at 4°C.

   - Formalin is not used as preservative for chemical analysis because extraction of poison, especially non-volatile organic compounds become difficult.

   - The use of disposable, hard plastic [especially polypropylene] or glass containers are recommended for preservation.

   - All samples should be properly sealed and labelled with the patient's name, hospital number, nature of sample, collection. It should be handed over to the IO after obtaining proper receipt.

- Sodium fluoride is the most commonly used agent to prevent glycolysis. It inhibiting bacterial growth.
- EDTA can effectively chelate the calcium ion of blood, therefore it can prevent the blood coagulation, does not affect the count and size of the leukocyte and keep erythrocyte invariable. Other anticoagulants are potassium oxalate, citrate or lithium heparin.

PROCEDURE OF PRESERVATION

For preservation of viscera, a clean, transparent and preferably sterile glass jar [one liter capacity] wide mouth and stoppers should be used. The size of the jar should be such that at least $1/3^{rd}$ of the container remains empty after being filled with the preservative to allow for accommodation of the gas which will evolve out of the organs preserved. However, the preservative should completely immerse the viscera after the contents are well shaken.

- The stomach, small intestine and its contents are preserved in one bottle, part of liver along with gallbladder, spleen and kidney in another bottle and urine in the third bottle. The stomach and intestines are opened before they are preserved. The liver and kidneys are cut into small pieces to ensure penetration of the preservatives. Blood should be sent in a vial.

- When additional material is required to be sent, it should be dispatched in separate bottles, like brain in one bottle. The bottles and vials required for preservation are normally supplied by the office of the Forensic science laboratory [FSL]

- The stoppers of the bottles should be well fitting, covered with a piece of cloth and tied by tape or string and the ends sealed using a department seal. Each bottle should be suitably labelled with the organ, date, time and place of autopsy, followed by signature of the doctor who performed the autopsy.

- A sample of the preservatives used [rectified spirit or sodium chloride] is separately preserved and sent for analysis to rule out any poison being present as a contaminant.

- The sealed bottles are then put in a viscera box which is sealed. A specimen of the seal used is put in a separate envelope which is sealed and handed over to the police constable, in return for a receipt. All these precautions are necessary to maintain the chain of evidence.

- Along with the viscera box, the following documents are also sent:
  I. Copy of inquest papers, brief facts of the case and case sheet.
  II. Copy of autopsy report.
  III. Letter requesting the chemical examiner to examine the viscera and inform the medical officer of its finding.[3]

NEGATIVE OR OBSCURE AUTOPSY

When the autopsy is completed, the medical officer must for an opinion as to the cause and manner of death and probable times since death. The abstract of this opinion should be given to the police constable accompanying the dead body for communication to the investigating officer. The information must include account of the decedent's history, description of the fatal environment, and circumstances surrounding death, the following are illustrative examples.[1]

I.   From the history of case and autopsy finding, I am of the opinion that this 50 year old man died due to haemorrhage from ruptured spleen as a result of a blow on the abdomen by the assailant.

II.   This 45 year old man died as a result of perforating gunshot wound of the head. Internal examination also called disclosed heart disease of the kind occasioned by a progressive narrowing of the coronary arteries. Information available at the time of examination combined with the finding of entry wound with visible powder residues on the root of the mouth support the conclusion that the manner of death was suicide.

III. These 50 years women died of coronary thrombosis. The automobile crash in which she was involved is believed to have the result of her death at the wheel. Laboratory examination of blood and tissues does not reveal; alcohol or other drugs.

The report should state the authority ordering the autopsy; name, age and sex of the deceased; date, place, and time of examination; and the means by which the body was identified. A complete description of external examination including detailed description of the injuries, their age, etc., is then given. Information about treatment is included when necessary. This is followed by a complete description of internal examination.

This part of the report contains details of positive findings, important negative findings, and general condition of other viscera. For instance, absence of airway obstruction, condition of the coronary arteries and heart valves, absence of pulmonary emboli, surgical absence of appendix, and the contents of stomach, gall bladder and urinary bladder, all merit inclusion. This is followed by conclusion as to the cause of manner of death, and approximate time elapsed since death, based as far as possible on post-mortem findings. Photographs, radiographs, sketch, weights, measurement, and laboratory reports provide an objective record and enhance the value of the autopsy report.

The opinion regarding the cause of the death is given in the form of a certificate filling up all its columns. This is followed by the signature, qualifications, and the designation of the medical officer.

The certificate about the cause of death is issued within 24 hours after conducting the autopsy. In case of poisoning, decomposed bodies, and/or when the cause of death requires further examination, e.g. chemical or microscopic, the opinion as to the cause of death is given when the result of such examination is known.

a) **CAUSE OF DEATH:** It is defined as a disease or injury or a combination of both that bought about cessation of life. When there is delay between the onset of a disease process or infliction of injury and the ultimate death of an individual, the proximate cause of death is the disease or injury that initiated a series of event that led directly to the immediate cause of death. Suppose a person dies of peritonitis two weeks after a stab in the abdomen. The immediate cause of death is peritonitis. The proximate cause of death is a stab wound of the abdomen. The physiological and biochemical disturbance, e.g. shock, sepsis, metabolic acidosis, ventricular fibrillation, respiratory arrest, etc., produced by the cause of death constitute the mechanism of death.

b) **MANNER OF DEATH:** This is expressed opinion based upon all available information of a particular case. This includes autopsy findings, laboratory reports, scene of death, medical history, etc. it can be classified as:

  I.   Natural – ischaemic heart disease
  II. Suicidal – incised wound on wrist, self-inflicted.
  III. Homicide – asphyxia by throttling [manual strangulation]
  IV. Accident – shock and haemorrhage due to multiple fractures, run over by a truck.
  V.   Undetermined [presumed natural] – unknown or unascertainable – no disease, no injury, no poisoning.

When there is no grossly discernible cause of death, histological examination should be including at least six sections of the heart to exclude myocarditis.[1]

OBSCURE AUTOPSY:

In about 20% of all post-mortem examination cases, the cause of death may not be clear at the time of dissection of the body and there are minimal or indeterminate findings or ever no positive findings at all. These are source of confusion to ant forensic pathologist.

It may of these cases, the cause of death can be made out after detailed clinical and laboratory investigation and interview with persons who had observed before he died.

Cause:-

  I.   Natural diseases – Epilepsy, paroxysmal fibrillation.
  II. Concealed trauma – Concussion, blunt injury to the heart, reflex vagal inhibition.
  III. Poisoning – Anaesthetic overdose, narcotic, neurotoxic, cytotoxic or plant poisoning.
  IV. Biochemical distribution – Uraemia, diabetes.
  V.   Endocrinal distribution – Adrenal insufficiency, thyrotoxicosis.
  VI. Endocrinal distribution – Allergy, drug idiosyncrasy.

NEGATIVE AUTOPSY:

In about 2-5% of all post-mortem examination cases, the cause of death remains unknown, even after all laboratory examinations including microscopic and toxicological examination.

Reasons of negative autopsy:-

I. Inadequate history.
II. Inadequate external examination and internal examination.
III. Insufficient laboratory examination.
IV. Lack of toxicological analysis.
V. Lack of training of the doctor.

SECOND AUTOPSY

There is no provision in Indian law for a second autopsy. Rarely, it is conducted either by order of the Magistrate or senior police officer by a border of doctors; usually three is number, from different institutions.

It is usually done when the relatives are not satisfied with the report given in the autopsy report or when the cause of death cannot be opined by the doctor in the first instance.[3]

FACTORS THAT INFLUENCE SUCH ESTIMATION

For investigation of crime, it is very important to determine time since death, also known as post-mortem interval [interval between death and the time of post-mortem examination]. It provides a clue to the investigating Officer to institute suitable inquiries to apprehend the persons likely to be responsible, and to estimate others from suspicion.

The point to estimate the approximate time since death includes:

I. Cooling of the body.
II. Post-mortem lividity
III. Rigor mortis
IV. Decomposition changes
V. Contents of the stomach and bowels
VI. Contents of urinary bladder
VII. Biochemical changes
VIII. Circumstantial evidence.

COOLING OF THE BODY:

A progressive fall in temperature is one of the most prominent early signs of death, the amount of cooling indicating the approximate time since death. The rate of cooling is not uniform but is related to the difference in temperature between the body and its surroundings. In a tropical country like India, the average heat loss is roughly 0.5° - 0.7°C per hour and the body attains environmental temperature in about 16-20 hours after death. However, if the environmental temperature is high, e.g. 40°C, the body temperature will go up [refer post-mortem caloricity].

POSTMORTEM LIVIDITY:

The incidence, extent, and degree of fixation of post-mortem lividity is important, it commences within an hour after death. Ina an average case of sudden death, it presents as a series of mottled patches over the dependent parts in about 1-3 hours. These patches coalesce in about 3-6 hours. The lividity is fully developed and fixed in about 6-8 hours. However, this is somewhat variable. **Lividity will not been seen;**

   a) If the body is constantly altering its position, e.g. in drowning
   b) If the skin is dark
   c) If much blood is lost e.g. in massive haemorrhage.

RIGOR MORTIS:

The presence and extent or absence of rigor mortis should be noted. In India, it usually commences in about 2-3 hours after death, takes about 12 hours to develop from head to foot, persists for another 12 hours, it takes 12 hours to pass off, in the same order in which it occurred. These timing are however subject to variation.

DECOMPOSITION CHANGES:

The presence, character and extent of putrefaction is very valuable indeed. In India, a greenish patch over the caecum and flanks appears in about 12-24 hours.it spreads over the whole of abdomen and the body within the next 24 hours.

Vascular marbling commences after 24 hours. Putrefactive odour is noticed at about the same time. By 36-48 hours, marbling is prominent.

In 12-18 hours, gases collect in the intestines and distend the abdomen. From 18 to 36 or 48 hours, gas formation is abundant. Gases collect in the tissues and hollow viscera, and accuse false rigidity and pressure effects. In about 36 hours after death in summer, the female genitals appear pendulous. In about 48-72 hours, the rectum and uterus protrude.

By about 18-36 hours, flies lay their eggs. The eggs hatch into maggots or larvae in about 24 hours. In the course of 4-5 days, maggots develop into pupae and, in another 4-5 days, pupae into adult flies. It should be remembered that eggs can laid even before death if the victim is debilitated or unconscious, the common sites being the wounds, and moist areas such as the eyelids, lips, nostrils, genitalia and anus.

In 3-7 days, teeth and sutures of skull in children and young adults become loose. In 5-12 days, soft tissues liquefy and break down. Only the more resistant viscera which putrefy in 2-3 weeks are discernible. In 1-3 months, the body is skeletonised.

The process of decomposition may be modified into adipocere formation or mummification.

The time required for adipocere formation in our country is 5-15 days, the shortest recorded being 3 days and 22 hours. The time required for complete mummification of a body varies from 3-12 months or longer.

CONTENTS OF THE STOMACH AND BOWEL:

The site and state of digestion of the contents of the stomach and bowel may be of some value in fixing the hour of death in relation to the last meal. Sometimes, the stomach content can be matched with a particular meal known to have been consumed.

The length of time required to empty the stomach after a meal is very variable, and depends on the type of meal ingested, stomach tome, pyloric function, and the psychological state of the individual. Fear and anxiety, for example, may cause great delay in the emptying rate, and power of digestion may remain suspended for a long time in conditions of shock and coma. Food has been seen in stomach remaining undigested in persons who received severe head injuries soon after their meal and died within 12-24 hours.

In general, milk leaves the stomach rapidly but the large vegetable meals consumed in India do not usually leave the stomach for at least 4 hours. Chapattis [bread] digest to a pulp fairly quickly, within about 2 hours, but do not leave the stomach quickly when other foods are present with them. Dals [pulses, lentils, beans] of all kinds retain their from upto 2 hours, and rice grains up to 3 hours. If meat has been eaten along with vegetable foods, it is seldom distinguishable as such after 3 hours, and after 4 hours both the green vegetables and roots are indistinguishable. In general, if at autopsy, one finds that the stomach is full, it would suggest that the victim died within 2 hours of talking the last meal if food was distinguishable, and 4 hours if it was indistinguishable.

Must be remembered that the process of digestion may not cease at death; the enzymes released may auto-digest the stomach wall resulting in perforation. Such an event, when found, males the state of food in the stomach an unreliable indicator of time since death even if the time and nature of the last meal are known.

The presence and absence of faeces in the large intestine mat be of some value. With most persons, it is customary to evacuate the bowel in the morning. If, therefore, the large intestine contains faeces, one may presume that death may have occurred sometime in the night, and if empty, sometime after evacuation in the morning.

CONTENTS OF THE URINARY BLADDER:

The amount of urine in urinary bladder may give some direction of the time since last micturition.

BIOCHEMICAL CHANGES:

Chemical constituents of CSF, such as lactic acid, non-protein nitrogen [NPN] and amino acid content increase in the first 15 hours after death but the rate is not uniform and is influenced by cooling of the body.

The potassium content of vitreous humour of the eye steadily rises after death. The range is, however, too wide. A progressive increase in levels of lactic acid, non-protein nitrogen, and certain enzymes, has also been observed after death, and this can be plotted graphically.

CIRCUMSTANTIAL EVIDENCE: This includes.

a) Growth of hair on face
b) Presence of lice hair
c) State of dress
d) Personal effects
e) Other data

Males generally shave the chin every day. Beard hair grows at the rate of 0.4 mm per day. From this, rough estimate may be made of the time since the last shave. Hair does not grow after death. The presence of lice is generally found on long hair of the head and infrequently even on short hair on other parts of the body. Lice generally die within 3-6 days of death of the individual. The state of dress, e.g., office dress or night dress may indicate the time of day that death has occurred. Personal effects, e.g., wrist watch, letters, daily, food, etc., all provide valuable data. If the body is in a room and lights and burning, it indicates that death occurred at night. If the body is lying on green grass [shrubs and plants], the grass becomes pale due to non-exposure to sun's rays about 5 days. Therefore, if pale grass is found under the body, it would suggest that death occurred more than 5 days ago.

A summary of important points is assessing time since death is appended in the table. It must be remembered that these times are average times in average circumstances and based on evaluation of general and individual variations; they apply to tropical climate; in cold weather, they may be doubled or trebled; and in the hills, they are quite inapplicable. It should also be remembered that these times refer to undisturbed and unmutilated body. Insects, birds, and wild animals, can skeletonise the body surprisingly quickly.

S.NO	Times since death	Condition of the body
1.	Less than 1 hour	Body warm.
2.	3 hours	Patchy post-mortem lividity.
3.	6-8 hours	Lividity fully developed and fixed
4.	12 hours	Rigor present all over. Green patches showing-over the caecum.
5.	24-36 hours	Body cold. Rigor receding/absent. Green discolouration over whole abdomen and spreading to chest. Abdomen distended with gases. Ova of flies seen.
6.	48 hours	Trunk bloated. Face discoloured and swollen.
7.	72 hours	Whole body glossy swollen and disfigured. Hair and nails loose. Tissues soft and discoloured.
8.	One week	Soft viscera putrefied
9.	Two week	Only the more resistant viscera distinguishable soft tissues largely gone
10.	1-3 months	Body skeletonised.[1]

EXAMINATION OF DECOMPOSED, MUTILATED AND SKELETONIZED REMAINS

- **Forensic anthropology** is that branch of physical anthropology which for forensic purposes deals with identification of skeletonized remains known to be or suspected to be being human.
- **Mass disaster:** Death of more than 12 victims in a single event, like fire, air crashes or flood. The number of victims far exceeds the capacity of local death investigation system of handle.

DECOMPOSED BODIES

Decomposed bodies show putrefactive changes in varying degree depending upon the time elapsed since death. In most cases, evidence of trauma (haemorrhage and fracture) can be recognized. Appropriate viscera should be preserved (whenever possible) for chemical analysis for evidence of suspected poisoning. [3]

The examination should be complete and should be held on the same lines as in ordinary autopsies. To save hard work on decomposed bodies and thus to lessen the chances of septic poisoning a pair of hooks made of ¼" iron or steel 9" long and with 3" bent in to form a handle is very convenient for hooking up the abdominal and other incisions so as to keep the part open and also for opening the pericardium and hooking up the heart, lungs and other organs.

In case of external fatal injuries it is not difficult to find out the cause of death.

In case of strangulation and hanging the cord mark would be apparent, even if the skin had peeled off, as the skin on and around about the mark persists for some time. In case of hanging Modi found a ligature mark in the neck on the sixth day after death when the body had been putrefied to a large extent.

The presence of mud in right bronchus at the post-mortem examination held on the fifth day after death when the body was advanced in putrefaction led Modi to form a diagnosis of drowning.

A foreign body, such as a bullet, a piece of a weapon or some other object, found in a body, may give a valuable clue to the cause of death.

In fracture of the skull bones disorganized clotted blood may be found on their inner plates, or on the surface of the Dura mater and on the brain in spite of its soft and pulpy nature if decomposition has not far advanced; but there mere effusion of blood on the brain would not be enough to warrant a statement that the fracture was caused before or after death. In doubtful cases a guarded opinion should be given that the injuries found on the body, if inflicted during the life, were sufficient to cause death and they might have been caused by such and such a weapon.

The necessary viscera should always be preserved foe chemical analysis in those cases where the cause of death cannot be found owing to advanced decomposition.[4]

MUTILATED BODIES AND FRAGMENTARY REMAINS

- **Mutilated bodies** are extensively disfigured, deprived of a limb or a part of the body, but the soft tissues, muscles and skin are still attached to the bones.
- **Fragmentary remains** include only fragments of the body such as head , trunk or limbs.[3]

A number of questions can be answered with ascending degree of completeness depending upon the type and condition of the material received for examination. The following information is especially liked for:

1. Source whether human or animal

2. If part belong to the same individual
3. Age
4. Sex
5. Stature
6. Race
7. Identity
8. Special features
9. Cause of death
10. Time since death

Source: this can be determined from knowledge of anatomy. In case of doubt, a part of the soft tissues, provided decomposition is not too far advanced, is sent in a dry condition and without adding any preservative to the forensic science laboratory for a precipitin test. The antiglobulin inhibition test is more sensitive than the precipitin test but requires more expertise.

In places situated near the medical colleges and anatomy dissection hells, part of human bodies, improperly disposed of, may be brought for examination; it is easy to determine their source from the dark colour, formalin odour, and the presence of red lead in the blood vessels and nutrient canals of bone.

If parts belong to the same individual: A mix-up of parts may occur in mass disasters.

The marts belong to same individual if they can be fitted to gather and there is no disparity or duplication. Testing for similarity of blood group and DNA from different parts is more conclusive.

Age: This can be determine from the state of epiphyses; state of teeth and lower jaw; calcification of laryngeal and sternal cartilages and hyoid bone; changes in sternum; closure of the cranial suture; condition of the symphyseal surface of the pubic bone; changes in the joint; and colour of the hair on the scalp, beard, moustache, and pubis. Histomorphometric methods based on correlation of the number of osteons per unit area of bone samples and age as established by researches and helpful.

Sex: The prostate and non-pregnant uterus resists putrefaction for a long period. Gross and microscopic examination of internal genitals, if available, is confirmatory. In their absence, the nature and character of the soft parts and configuration of pelvis are helpful. If only the head is received, sex can be surmised from the presence or absence or bread. Sex can also be determined by nuclear sexing or sexing root sheath cells of head hair.

Stature: This is already discussed in the chapter on 'Identification in mass disaster'.

Race: This can be determined from hair and skin, if available, and from nasal bridge height, nasal aperture shape, facial prognathism, palate shape, incisors, the skull (cephalic index), pelvis, etc.

Identity: This can be determine from fingerprint, dental status, and personal property or articles in close proximity to the body. Also helpful are the congenital features like moles and acquired peculiarities like tattoo marks, condition of the palms, scars, deformities, and amputation marks. Evidence of any disease, e.g. gall stones, uterine fibroids, and appendectomy scar when present, is corroborative. Determination of blood group antigens A, B and H from teeth pulp might help to establish identity if the blood group is known. Selected X-Rays, dental X-Rays, and/or total body X-Ray are helpful if antemortem X Rays are available for comparison.

Special features: Mutilation may be the work of
1. Persons with anatomical knowledge
2. Other without such knowledge
3. Animals
4. May result from decomposition changes

Each has its own characteristics and therefore the manner in which the parts are mutilated is quite important.

Persons with anatomical knowledge destroy identifying features, as in the well-known Ruxton case. Others without such knowledge disfigure the body haphazardly, as for example, by use of saw, axe, or any heavy weapon. Animals generally attack the exposed parts and produce ghastly wounds resembling haphazard mutilation; however, careful examination will reveal if the bones are gnawed through by animals or cut by sharp weapons. In addition, animals generally eat away the medulla of long bones and spicules of cortical bone are found depressed in the medullary cavity. A separation of the body parts is brought about by decomposition also. The natural sequence is: soft parts, articular cartilages, and ligaments. Separation of joints of the hyoid as a result of decomposition may be mistaken for fracture.

Cause of death: An opinion as to the cause of death is possible when there is some evidence of antemortem violence such as injury to some large blood vessel or some vital organ, or the recovery of a bullet. It must however be remembered that mutilated fragments of the body decompose quickly and antemortem changes disappear or become indistinguishable from post-mortem ones. Sometimes, there may be some clues as a depressed fracture of the skull, fracture of hyoid, fracture-dislocation of cervical vertebra, severe injury to bones by a cutting instrument, or fractures of several ribs.

Sometimes, chemical examination of the available material for evidence of poisoning may also help. Obvious signs of disease such as a malignant growth of soft tissues, bones, etc., should be looked for.

Time since death: The probable time since death can be ascertained from the condition of the soft parts in relation to the process of putrefaction.[1,5]

BONES

A complete list of bones received for examination is prepared preferably along with the photograph of each bone. The bones are cleaned if necessary, then arranged in the normal anatomical manner, and the reconstruction skeleton photographed.

The scheme for the examination of bones is similar to that for mutilated bodies. An anatomist, dentist, anthropologist, and radiologist with medicolegal experience should be consulted. An opinion can be given on the following aspect:

1. Source, whether human or animal
2. Belong to one or more individuals
3. Age
4. Sex
5. Stature
6. Race
7. Identity
8. Special features
9. Cause of death
10. Time since death.

Source: This can be determined from
I.   Gross anatomical characteristics of human and animal bones
II.   Microscopic characteristics,
III. Chemical analysis of bone ash. In case of doubt, precipitin test may settle the issue.

One or more individuals: This can be determined from the number of bones received from the examination, noting the side to which they belong, and checking, for their fitting, duplicate, and morphological similarities. For example, if a skull belongs to the female aged about 18 years, other parts should also be of a female about that age. Similarly, there can be only one right humerus. However, supernumerary ribs, toes, and fingers must be borne in mind. If a mix-up of bones is suspected, they can be subjected to short wave ultraviolet lamp to separate them by the difference in colour emission.

Age: This can be determined from state of epiphyses; state of teeth, and lower jaw, calcification of laryngeal and sternal cartilages and hyoid bone; changes in sacrum; closure of cranial sutures; condition of symphyseal surface of pubic bone; changes in joints; histological examination of teeth; and cross section of mid-shaft area of femur, tibia or fibula.

Stature: This can be calculated if a long bone such as femur, tibia, humerus, or radius is available in its entirety, using the formulae of Dupertius and hadden and trotter and glesser for Americans; breitinger of Germans; telkka for Finns; and multiplication factors devised by Indian workers for Indians. While applying the various formulae, due account needs to be taken of the sex and race of the deceased by reference to appropriate tables. However, the following data provide a simple means to estimate the stature of a person. In general, humerus represents 20%, tibia 22%, femur 27%, and the spine 34% of the stature.

Race: An expert can determine this is a high proportion of cases from an examination of skull, mandible and teeth, pelvis, and lime bones.

Identity: Malunited fractures, healing fractures, or deformities of bone, when present, are helpful. When the skull is available, superimposition photography and facial reconstruction may be attempted. An X-Ray of any bone taken during life may be compared with an X-Ray of the same bone. Determination of blood group antigens A, B, and H from teeth pulp might also help in establishing identity if the blood group is known. DNA profiling also helps. It may be possible to obtain material for blood grouping and DNA profiling from cancellous bone.

Special features: by a meticulous examination of the ends of long bones, one can determine if the bones are cut by a sharp instrument or sawn through, or whether they are gnawed through by animals and medulla eaten away. In bones that are gnawed through, spicules of cortical bone will be found depressed into the medullary cavity.

Cause of death: this is difficult to determine unless there are some clues. Fractures, especially of skull, hyoid, ribs, and other bones, should be looked for; knife scratches on clavicle vertebral bodies and other bone or joint surface, if found, are informative. An opinion on these features however is difficult sine the antemortem evidence disappears rapidly after death. A foreign body, such as a bullet when present in a bone, is helpful. Bones or their charred remains may be subjected to chemical analysis for the detection of metallic poisons, such as arsenic, as these are not destroyed by heat. Neutron activation analysis technique helps to detect certain metallic poisons in quantities far below the limits of conventional analysis. Maggots may reveal the presence of drugs.

Time since death: This is also difficult to estimate. Bodies exposed on the ground may be skeletonised even in a day if attacked by animals. However, an inference can be drawn from the following:

In the process of skeletisation, soft tissues disappear first, then articular cartilages, and finally ligaments. In case of a fracture, examination of the callus after dissecting it longitudinally may give some clues as regards time. Bones are foul smelling and humid in recent cases (about 1-3 months). When they undergo putrefaction, they lose organic matter and therefore become light and fragile. Old bones tend to be dry, light, fragile, and the marrow cavity is also dry, and free of fat.

HANDLING OF HIV INFECTED AND HEPATITIS B POSITIVE BODIES

HIV infection should be suspected if the body is of

I.   A male homosexual

II.   An intravenous drug abuser

III.   A haemophiliac who has received repeated blood transfusions

IV.   A female prostitute,

V.   A victim of sex abuse

The staff should be vaccinated against hepatitis B and re-vaccinated at intervals when the antibody titre falls below protective level. At every stage, care should be taken to avoid direct contact of skin and mucous membrane with body fluid and tissues. Hands should be washed thoroughly with soap and water after each activity even if gloves are worn.

Special precautions are necessary at each stage, viz

I.   At the scene

II.   In the autopsy room

III.   In the laboratory

IV.   On the court, in addition to

V.   General precautions.

AT THE SCENE

I.   Disposal shoe protection by persons at the scene is necessary.

II.   Food or smoking should not be allowed at the scene.

III.   Blood-contaminated clothing or other material should be handled carefully. Dried blood or wet blood material that is not to be stored as evidence should be decontamination and properly disposal off by incineration.

IV.   Non-disposable material used during the investigation and collection of evidence at the scene should be decontaminated by usual hypochlorite solution.

IN THE AUTOPSY ROOM

I. Admission: No unauthorised person should be admitted to the autopsy and body preparation room.

II. Clothing: protection includes complete covering of the body be wearing double gloves, gowns, water-proof aprons, caps, masks, goggles if eye glasses are not worn, and shoe-cover.

III. Instruments: minimum instruments as required should be kept. At the start of the autopsy, a knife, scalpel, scissors and forceps are kept to start with. Scissor with slightly blunted points should be routinely used and the small sharp ones only when needed. Special care is necessary to handle sharp items such as needles and scalpels to prevent accidental pricks and cuts.

IV. Disposal requirements: Instruments, working surfaces used in the procedure, associated gloves, protective clothing, and waste material must be disinfected, sterilised, or incinerated as appropriate.

V. Handling specimens for laboratory examination: Gloves should be worn at all times by laboratory as well as autopsy room and mortuary personnel when handling specimens from suspected cases.

VI. Clean up procedure: New intact disposable gloves should be worn. Small spatters and spills of blood and other body fluids can be wiped up with disposable tissues or towels which are discarded in special bio-hazard bags and properly disposed off, and the area then covered with a disinfectant and wiped clean.

VII. Disinfection: A 1:10 dilution of household bleach or a freshly prepared sodium hypochlorite solution, the active ingredient in the bleach, in equivalent concentration of 5000 ppm, is recommended.

VIII. Accidental injury and prophylaxis: In the event of an accidental injury, contaminated or not with bloody and body fluids, either at autopsy or in the laboratory, the wound should be disinfected and the incident report to the proper authority. Blood sample should be taken from the source of exposure and tested for HIV and hepatitis B. Blood sample should be taken from the injured person for immediate testing and for comparison during the follow up period. The test should be repeated at 6 weeks, 3 months, 6 months, and 1 year after episode. Any person who is accidentally exposed to HIV should have a prophylactic course of Zidovudine, 500 mg twice a day, for 6 weeks. Any person exposed to hepatitis B and who is not vaccinated should have prophylactic hepatitis B immunoglobulin within 72 hours of the incident, followed by active vaccination.

IN THE LABORATORY

I.   Disposable gloves should be worn and counter top covers used in areas where biological material is examined. This should be disposed off in an authorised manner.

II.   Food or smoking should not be allowed in the work area.

III.   All biological specimens should be considered contaminated and treated accordingly.

IV.   Mouth-pipetting of biological material should not be allowed.

V.   If possible, specimens to be destroyed should be burnt or chemically decontaminated.

VI.   Hands should be washed before leaving the work area.

IN THE COURT

I.   Whenever possible, biological contaminated evidence should be referred by photographic or other means rather than presenting it in court.

II.   When necessary bullets, clothing, etc., should be handled using disposable gloves and over paper, or the (dry-not wet/moist) evidence should be enclosed in a sealed, clear, plastic bag.

III.   The hands should be washed after handling the evidence.

GENERAL PRECAUTIONS

The best key to control the dissemination of HIV or hepatitis B is prevention – prevention of unnecessary contamination of the work area and of injuries. Prevention required strict attention to details, carrying out the required autopsy and body preparation procedures with care, neatly and cleanly, avoiding spattering and confining any flow of body fluids within limited bounds of the work area.

The major danger to all personnel would be any action the produces an aerosol of biological material, such as that produced by a saw during autopsy or by a blender in toxicology studies. The most common known methods of accidental exposure include being pricked with a used needle or other contaminated material, and the contamination of an area or surface, which would not be expected to be so, by the thoughtless techniques of a careless fellow employee. Washing hands and cleaning floors, doors, door knobs, and telephone with a disinfectant capable to killing viruses will protect the employees.[1,5]

Referances:

1. Parikh's Textbook of Medical Jurisprudence, Forensic Medicine and Toxicology (sixth edition) by –C.K.Parikh, Sixth edition reprint - 2012 by Cbs Publishers & Distributors Pvt. Ltd.

2. Hand book of forensic medicine and toxicology by S.C. BASU, Edited by –A. K. Gupta

3. Forensic Medicine and Toxicology Including Clinical and Pathological Aspects (SECOND EDITION) by – Gautam Biswas, published by – Jaypee Brothers Medical Publishers (P) Ltd

4. MODI'S MEDICAL AND JURISPRUDENCE AND TOXICOLOGY by – N. J. Modi, 23rd Edition by – Tripathi.

5. Krishan Vij Textbook of Forensic medicine and Toxicology, 4th Edt.

Chapter 4

THANATOLOGY

Thanatology Greek, thanatos-death, Logos-science] is the branch of medical science that studies death with all its aspects. The term death is commonly employed to denote 'the cessation of life in the body as whole. 'As per registration of birth and deaths act 1969, section 2(b), death is the permanent disappearance of all the evidence of life at any time after live birth has taken place.

A person who has sustained either;

- 1. Irreversible cessation of circulatory and respiratory functions, or
- 2. Irreversible cessation of all the functions of the entire brain, including the brainstem, is dead. Determination of death, which has tremendous social and legal importance, must be made in accordance with accepted medical standards.

Types of death;

Death is of two types.

- Somatic or clinical or systemic death.
- Molecular or cellular death (few minutes to hours).

Signs of death;

- Signs of somatic death (immediate / clinical and continuous) of circulation for more than 5 minutes.
- Absolute cessation (complete and continuous of respiration for more than 5 minutes.
- Absolute cessation (complete and continuous) of central Nervous system functions or brain death for at least 5 minutes.

Signs of molecular death;

1. Change in the eyes (dilated fixed pupils etc.)
2. Changes in the skin (loss of elasticity).
3. Complete loss of temperature and cooling of the body.
4. Cadaveric lividity or post-mortem staining of hypostasis or suggillation.
5. Rigor mortis or cadaveric rigidity.
6. Secondary relaxation or flaccitidy.
7. Putrefaction or decomposition (bluish-green discolouration of front of right lower abdomen,- earliest and surest sign).
8. Saponification or adipocere.
9. Mummification

Death in absence of saponification, mummification or intrauterine maceration.

Following features are examined to certify death clinically.

1. Absence of pulse in the peripheral arteries (e.g., brachial artery at the elbow and carotid on front of neck).
2. Absence of heart sound on auscultation. Flat (isoelectric) E.C.G or cessation of heart's activity on a cardiac monitor.
3. Absolute Cessation of Respiration;
4. Absence of respiratory movement of chest on inspection and breath sound on auscultation.
5. Absolute cessation of CNS function
6. Absence of corneal reflex and jerks and primary flaccidity of muscles.
7. No response to ordinary painful stimuli (pin prick).

Suspended animation or Death trance

Stoppage of circulation and respiration not be relied upon as absolute signs of death, because patients have stopped as was evident from clinical examination.

This is called Suspended animation (Death trance); i.e. the three vital functions of life

(Animation) have been rebuked (suspended) to be is in a transitional zone between life and death. This is said to be practices by Yogis (voluntary death trance); it may be rarely seen in persons suffering from Hysteria. Involuntary death trance is seen in New born, Cholera, Electrocution, Narcotic poisoning Anesthetic shock Sun-stroke, Concussion, Drowning, Hanging, Tetanus acute Convulsions, and in Severe shock. This stage may last from a few seconds to half an hour or more. These cases can sometimes be revived by external cardiac massage, electric stimulation of heart and artificial respiration. Attending doctor should act promptly and start treatment without animation, it should be reported to local police station for making necessary arrangement for medico legal post-Mortem Examination to avoid possible charges of Medical Negligence and diagnosis of actual cause of death.[1,2,3,4,5,6,7]

Moment of Death

Following tests should be undertaken before death is announced by doctor for cadaver Organ Trans-plantation and removal of Heath-Lung machines or Cardiac, Lung and other monitors to use for another dying patient.

(i) Rectal temperature - below 24degree Celsius

(ii) Ophthalmoscopy– reveals segmentation of retinal blood columns.

(iii) Absence of electrical activities in EEG, i.e. isoelectric EEG for five minutes. (Most important sing that is regarded as the Moment of death).

Some developing countries of this world do not honour the significance of diagnosis of moment over the dead body to the relatives four hours after Clinical Certification of death i.e. after well developed Rigor mortis is seen all over the body i.e. after molecular death i.e. Rigor mortis etc. has set in[1-8].

STUDY OF MOLECULAR DEATH SIGNS

Following signs or changes are studied:

CHANGES IN EYES

1. Loss of intraocular tension of eyeballs.
2. Loss of luster of eyes.
3. Cornea-opaque, hazy or cloudy. It becomes soft and pits on pressure. If cornea is kept moist with saline,it may remain transparent for some time when an ophthalmoscopic examination may reveal fragmentation of blood columns in retinal vessels with blurring of macula and margin of optic disc.
4. Techenoir sclerotica or brownish black discolouration of sclera and conjunctive is seen in partly open eyelids for 2 to 3 hours after death.
5. Shape of the pupil is round in a living person, but by pressing the eyeballs of dead persons by fingers, one can change the shape of pupil as muscle of Iris has lost its power.
6. But pupils will react to myotic (physostignine) or mydriatic (atropine) for 1 to 2 hours after death (till molecular death sets in).
7. Potassium level in vitreous humour rises with time passed after death.
8. Softening of eyeball occurs by 6-12 hours in summer.

CHANGES IN SKIN

1. Loss of lustre.
2. Loss of elasticity; incised wound produced after death will not gape much and contact flattening over back and buttock, pinched up skin will not return to normal position promptly etc.
3. Changes in the colour; it becomes pale or ashy white.
4. Lips ; dry, brownish

LOSS OF TEMPERATURE AND COOLING OF BODY

As soon as life departs, the body at once commences to lose its heat, by conduction, convection and radiation because oxidation, which maintains body heat, has stopped. The body assumes the temperature of medium in which it is placed. Normal body temperature of surrounding is 37 deg C while mean temperature of surrounding is 30 deg C. That is the difference between body temperature and atmospheric temperature is not much in tropical climate. Average rate of cooling is 0.4 deg C per hour. With in 24 hours the body becomes as cold as its surrounding in temperate climate. In India on account of little difference of two temperatures, the body comes to the temperature of surroundings much earlier (about 12-15 hours). When this is plotted on a graph paper a sigmoid curve is seen. Rate of cooling of body (algor mortis) is hastened or delayed according to following circumstances.[5,6,7,8]

POST- MORTUM CALORICITY;

The term is used where the body temperature instead of coming down to normal room temperature after death, shows a slight rise of temperature which persists for an hour or two. This may happen in Tetanus, Cholera, Smallpox (earlier), Rheumatic fever, Liver abscess , Injury to nervous system Sunstroke, Strychnine poisoning and cerebrospinal meningitis. This post-mortem rise of temperature is due to the actions of micro-organisms in living tissues and fluids of the body and muscular contraction and defective heat regulating centre prior to death. Increase in heat production as seen in convulsion due to muscular over activity also contributes to a large extent.

CADAVERIC LIVIDITY

(POST-MORTEM STAINING)

This is also known as hypostasis or suggillation or livor mortis. This happens after the stoppage of heart's action or circulating; the fluid blood obeying the law of gravity, tends to go down into the capillaries of the most dependent parts of the body at that particular position and causes distension of the minute capillaries. This is show externally on the skin surface as purplish red areas of discoloration except over the parts pressed upon or flattened by contact with surface, thus causing compression of the capillaries and preventing them from being filled with fluid blood.

This is also seen in the internal tissues and organs, which have occupied the most dependent position after the death i.e posterior cerebral lobe of brain, posterior surfaces of the lungs, heart, liver, kidneys and posterior wall of the stomach and dependent parts of coils of small intestine. This is called Internal Hypostasis; blood remains fluid for 4-5 hours may be 6 hours after death. During this time alteration of position will change the position of post-mortem staining; but the area of post-mortem staining does not shift six hours after death. So, this gives an idea, about the time passed after the death and whether position of the body was altered after death(i.e , with in 4 to 6 hours).

In some cases, it may go on upon 10 to 12 hours, if the blood remains fluid, which is possible, in deaths due to violent asphyxia. In case of death due to massive haemorrhage (e.g. cut throat injury). Post-mortem staining will be poorly manifested; it is almost absent in severely anaemic subjects.

Post-mortem staining depends upon the character of Haemoglobin and fluidity of blood. In disseminated intravascular clotting, post-mortem staining may not appear. Hypostatic congestion may occur in week, asthenic and debilitated subjects, a few minutes before their death, owing to the feeble and slow circulation on dependent parts. This stained portion would remain so long the body does not get putrefied[8,9].

MEDICOLEGAL IMPORTANCE;

    i.   Reliable sign of death.

   ii.   May indicate time passed, since death.

  iii.   Gives information about the position of the body at the time of death and whether it has been altered or not.

  iv.   Indicates the cause of death from is colour (dusky red-normal). i.e. colour of Haemoglobin.

      1.   Bluish violet or purple in asphyxia.

2. Cherry red or pink in CO2, CO, CN and colubrine type of snake poisoning.

3. Chocolate in KCIO3, OR potassium bichromate poisoning.

4. Dark brown in phosphorus poisoning.

5. Jelly red in cases of death due to burns, because a large amount of smoke is inhaled.

UNSTAINED AREAS GIVING FALSE IMPRESSION;

Post-mortem staining will be absent from those parts which have been compressed by tight clothing or tight wrapping of sheet and these pale areas seen as stripes or bands called vibices, which often resemble the marks produced by flogging. Similarly, a white band on the neck produced by a tight callor a white band of the skin above may look like a ligature marks of strangulation.

If the head is turned to one side, the skin of the dependent side is thrown into folds. In these folds, the skin is under a certain degree of pressure and therefore, no stains can form.

Post-mortem stain and Congestion

Sometimes post-mortem staining on internal organ may be mistaken for congestion of it. Following points are to observed for correct diagnosis.

1. Congestion is uniform and involves the whole of the particular organ instead of its dependent portion which is usually affected by post-mortem staining

2. The mucosa in case of post-mortem staining becomes dull.

3. Inflammatory exudates will be evident in congestion while there may be alternate red and pale areas, when a hollow viscus, affected by post-mortem stain is examined in front of a light.

CONTACT FLATTENING AND POST-MORTEM STAINING'

During the period of primary flaccidity of muscles the soft convex portions of the body, e.g., scapula, buttocks, scalp and calf region which lie in contact with a hard surface, becomes flat from pressure. Post-mortem staining is absent in areas of contact flattening.

CADAVERIC CHANGES IN MUSCLES;

Immediately after death, all the muscles of the body become flaccid. Lower jaw falls, while limbs are perfectly mobile and muscle response to electrical stimuli. The muscles pass through three distinct phases.

1. Primary Relaxation or flaccidity with contractibility (first phase).- somatic death.

2. Complete rigidity, but no contractibility (second phase).- molecular death.

3. Secondary flaccidity or relaxation without contractibility (third phase).- molecular death.

Molecular death is manifested by stiffening or rigidity of all of muscles-involuntary and voluntary.

Followed by secondary flaccidity:

- First stage or the stage of flaccidity (primary relexation).
  Extremities are soft and flabby, joints are relaxed. But the muscles are contractile to external stimulus. It is the sign of somatic death. It may last commonly for 1 to 2 hours after death (average duration in India).

- Second stage (Rigor mortis)
  It begins after first stage and take 1 hours 56 minutes (within 1-2 hours after death in India) to be fully established. Once the body has become stiff, the body remains as such for 19 hours 12 minutes(roughly, total duration is 24 hours).
  But average duration of rigor mortis in temperate climate is 48 hours, and northern India it is24-48 hours, shorterst period for period for

rigor mortis to develop is 3hours. With the lapse of 19 hours 12 minutes (Bengal) muscles again become soft and the body enters into the third stage i.e, stage of secondary relaxation.

- Third stage (secondary relaxation)
  After rigor mortis the body again becomes soft and flaccid but does not respond to electrical stimulus. Third stage coincides sometimes with beginning of decomposition.

RIGOR MORTIS

It is the post-mortem contracted state of muscle with some degree of shortening of fibres. Rigor mortis first appears in the involuntary muscles of the body e.g heart and then in the voluntary group.

Orbicularis oculi is the first voluntary muscle involved. The heart is affected an hour after death. Post-mortem delivery may occur owing to the contraction of the uterine muscle. Earlier it comes on, more quickly it disappears. Longer it takes to appear, longer it persists. The rigor mortis, which is also known as a cadaveric rigidity of muscles, follows a definite order as it appears in the voluntary muscles.

PROXIMO-DISTAL ORDER OF APPEARANCE;

Rigor mortis appears in voluntary muscles in following order;

i.   Eyelid, lower jaw and face.

ii.   Muscles of the back of the neck and trunk.

iii. Upper limbs, front of the neck and chest.

iv.   Muscles of abdomen and lower limbs.
     It disappears also in the same order with the commencement of third stage of cadaveric changes is muscles.

MECHANISM;

The principal factors concerned in maintaining suppleness or plasticity of muscle protein i.e, actin and myosin filaments which remain separated. This hydration is dependent on the amount of ATP which is absorbed into proteins of the muscles. At the somatic death enough ATP is present in the muscle to maintain suppleness. After death, ATP gradually decomposes and is broken down to ADP, dehydration of muscles takes place and this result in interdigitation of Actin and Myosin filaments , this condition known as ' Rigor Mortis'. Subsequent relaxation (i.e, 3rd stage of cadaveric changes of muscle) is due to final decomposition of muscle with onset of putrefaction.

Stiffness in rigor mortis is closely related to the coagulation of muscles plasma and formation of lactic acid, which accumulates in the muscles. The reaction of muscle during the stage of rigor mortis is acidic while in the third stage, consequent upon decomposition of actomyosin, the reaction again becomes altered.

At the time of onset of putrefaction, there is breaking down of actomyosin complex of muscles fibres.

MEDICOLEGAL IMPORTANCE OF RIGOR MORTIS;

1. It is a dependable sign of death.
2. It gives information about Time of Death and sometimes mode of death.
3. It gives information about position of the body at the time of death unless already disturbed.

CONDITIONS STIMULATING RIGOR MORTIS;

1. Cadaveric spasm.
2. Heat stiffening – hardening or stiffening of muscle owing to coagulation of muscle albumin by heat. This is seen in death due to burns or when a body is suddenly dipped into the boiling fluid. The temperature must exceed 65 deg C. Rigor mortis does not develop; in muscles affected by

rigor mortis. Pugilistic attitude- attitude of a boxer in defence taken up by the body in death due to heat stiffening.

3. Cold stiffening- Here muscles are stiff due to solidification of fat and freezing of body fluid due to extreme cold. This stiffening rapidly disappears in contact with warmth and rigor mortis appears.

4. Gas stiffening or putrefaction Inflation of tissues by putrefactive gas.

CADAVERIC SPASM (INSTANTANEOUS RIGOR)

This is a phenomenon in which muscles that have been in a state of contraction during last part of life, become stiff and rigid immediately after death without passing through the initial stage of relaxation. Hence, attitude of the body, adopted at the time of death maintained for several hours after the death and its continuous with the rigidity that sets in other muscles after death. It is the continuation of the contraction of the muscles after death. The contraction of muscles is the result of nervous influence, when there is great muscular exertion and mental excitement before death. This is may be observed in voluntary muscle in death from Tetanus, Hydrophobia, Strychnine poisoning, concussion in children, sudden violent asphyxia death as in drowning and hanging[2,3,5,6]

References:

1. Basu S.C., Hand Book Of Forensic Medicine and Toxicology, third edition (2007), Current Distributors, Lenin Saranee, Calcutta.(page no. 1,3-10).
2. Mahanta Putul, Modern Textbook of Forensic Medicine And Toxicology (2014), Jaypee Brothers Medical Publishers, Darya Ganj, New Delhi. (Page no. 8-13,16,17,20).
3. Parikh C.K., Parikh's textbook of medical jurisprudence forensic medicine and toxicology, sixth edition (2011),C.B.S. Publishers and Distributors, Ansari Road, Darya Ganj, New Delhi. (Page no. 1.3,1.4,1.9,1.17,1.19).
4. Kumar Avinash, Law Of Evidence, third edition (2011), Singhal Law Publications, Burari, Delhi -84. (P.105,106,130,172,176,177,178,209,216).
5. Modi. Jaising. P, Textbook of Medical Jurisprudence And Toxicology, Twenty First Edition (1997), N.M. Tripathi Private Limited, Bombay.

6.   Usmani Hammad, Tib-Ul-Qanoon, First edition (1976), Universal Book House, Allahabad. (P.17-33).
7.   www.wikipedia.com
8.   Krishan Vij Textbook of Forensic medicine and Toxicology, 4th Edt.

Chapter 5

PUTREFACTION (DECOMPOSITION)

PUTREFACTION (DECOMPOSITION)

Putrefaction is a process by which complex organic matters of the body are transformed into simple inert inorganic matters.

Putrefaction is usually seen when rigor mortis disappears. It is the most absolute and surest sign of death. Putrefaction occurs as results of activity of a variety of organisms-aerobic and anaerobic bacteria normally present in the large bowel in human being principal offender is Cl. Welchii.

Shortly after death they invade into the blood stream from the bowel. Richly vascular organs or those in proximity from the source of bacteriae are putrefied first.

These bacteriae liberate various proteolytic, saccharolytic and lipolytic enzymes destroy various tissues. Lecithinase from Cl. Welchii dissolves the lecithin of cell membranes including those of RBC and cause post-mortem haemolysis. In our country, disappearance rigor mortis and onset decomposition are usually present at the same time, specially during summer seasons.

STAGE OF PUTREFACTION

As per Mackeneie following sign of decomposition are seen hourwise after death in Wet Bengal.

COLOUR CHANGES

It is usually noted by 24 to 36 hours after death in summer and 36 to 48 the skin over the right iliac region of abdomen except in case of drowning where this may be first seen on the skin of the face, front of the neck, or that of the upper part of chest.

Iliac region of abdomen is affected first on account of proximity of the caecum, where putrefactive organisms reside in large numbers. By 12-18 hours it may spread all over the abdomen in summer (India). In dextroposition of the viscera the colour change will first occur in the left side lower abdomen.

CAUSE

Change of colour is due to a change in the blood pigment from liberation of H_2S from the decomposed tissues and its combination with methaemoglobin obtained from Hb of broken down RBC, to from sulph-meth-haemoglobin (bluish-green in colour).

Skins of back neck, chest, upper limbs, scrotum and lower limbs become greenish. Superficial veins of skin are seen through the skin as dark, irregular purplish streaks near axillae, grain and adjoining areas of chest and thigh. This is known as Marbling and is commonly seen 36 to 48 hours after death.

FOUL SMELL

This appears by 36-48 hours after death depending on environmental temperature. Owing to the formation of foul smelling gases due to decomposition of tissues, body emits a disagreeable bad odour.

EFFECTS OF COLLECTION OF GAS

Gases collect in the soft tissues and cavities, abdomen swells up. The subcutaneous tissues feel spongy, especially where their texture is loose as in the neck and scrotum. As a result of considerable pressure within, features are distorted and may not be recognisable. Face is bloated eyeballs and tongue protrude. Lips swell and become everted. Frothy blood stained fluid from lungs contents of stomach are forced out of mouth. On account of distension of abdomen, their is pressure on the blood vessels to drive there blood into the heart and lungs. The gases cause anus to gape and faeces are expelled. The rectum and uterus may prolapsed. Postmortem delivery may take place with or without inversion of the uterus. Later on weight of all organs decrease in highly decomposed dead bodies.

POST-MORTEM EMPHYSEMA

Inflation of the decomposed body by the putrefaction gases leading to gross alteration of the features. It is known as post-mortem Emphysema.

POST-MORTEM BLISTERS

They appear usually 36-72 hours after death, average 49 hours 34 mins. The cuticles are raised into bullae or blister. Antemortem blister due to burns have red line around the blisters and it contains serum with high albumin content. The postmortem blisters contain mainly gas and small amount of reddish coloured fluid, poor in albumin contents and can be peeled off easily. Bruises are now difficult to recognize. If there is any wound, it gives a false impression of bleeding from the wound due to the pressure of the gas within the vessels. This is called post-mortem bleeding.[1,2,3,4,5.]

MAGGOTS

Flies attracted by the foul smells (by 36 to 48 hours)begin to lay their eggs on various parts of dead bodies, particularly in open wound, natural orifices and moist areas (axilla and groin). The eggs hatch into maggots (immature) or larvae in another 18 to 24 hours in hot weather. Maggots crawl into the interior of the body and help in destroying soft tissues and eat them up and develop into mature maggots; the maggots produce holes which may be wrongly diagnosed as Gunshot wounds. Sometimes, maggots may appear before death on neglected or undressed and infected ulcers and gangrenous areas.

Maggots become pupae in 4-5 days and pupae leave the dead body and go to earth developed into adults flies in other 3-5 days. If body is kept in a tightly closed room where flies cannot enter or it is covered with a fresh cloth nicely, no maggots can develop. Sometimes, immature maggots may appear by 24 hours 57 minutes and maggots may appear maggots by 39 hours 43 minute. In warm climates, maggots appear much earlier than in cold environment.

SEPARATION OF SOFT PARTS

This occurs 3-5 days after death. Nails and hairs become loose and can be easily peeled off or detached. Degloving of skin of palm and destocking of soles of feet also occur. Sutures of skull specially in children, give way and liquefied brain runs out. Abdomen and thorax soften, burst open and all soft tissues and organs are now converted into a thick, semifluid, black mass. The soft tissues ultimately fall off exposing the bare bones of the skeleton.

Skeletonisation take 7-10 days to occur under water where various aquatic animals eat the flesh and in similar period if a body is kept unburied and exposed to vultures and wild animals. Buried body take about a year to become completely skeletonised. Obviously, mediumin which the body is placed determines the skeletonisation time. After some years bones are even destroyed.

Colliquative putrefaction – hairs, nails, teeth and bones remain unaltered for a long time and they help in identification of the body and determination cause of death (poisoning).

PUTREFACTION OF INTERNAL ORGANS

Side by side with decomposition of external structures, internal organs also show putrefaction. Some organs putrefy rapidly and some organs putrefy rapidly and some late.

ORGANS PUTREFYING RAPIDLY

1. Larynx and trachea (onset of decomposition of these organs almost coincide with the discolouration of the right iliac region of abdomen).
2. Brain of a child.
3. Intestine and stomach.
4. Spleen.
5. Liver (honey-comb appearance).

142

6. Brain of adult.

7. Pregnant or puerperal uterus.

ORGANS PUTREFYING LATER

1. Heath.

2. Lungs.

3. Kidneys.

4. Urinary bladder.

5. Pancreas.

6. Blood vessels.

7. Uterus of virgin

8. Prostate.

   The virgin uterus and prostate can be recognized even 6-7 months after the death in some cases and help in the identification of sex of a highly decomposed unknown subject.

RATE OF PUTREFACTION[6]

These depend on three media, in which a dead body can be kept, i.e.,

- Air
- Under water
- Buried under the earth.

1. Rate of putrefaction also varies as follows : if this rate in air is considered to be 1, it will be ½ of that in the water , and $1/8^{th}$ of that under the earth. But a drowned body, when recovered from water and brought to land (air) will show very quick onset of putrefaction. It will be 14 times its original rate in water (i.e., 7 time the usual land rate due to imbibation of water).

2. Putrefaction starts very rapidly if body is lying in polluted water which contains large number of bacteriae.

3. Wounded bodies also putrefy quickly. In multilated bodies different parts putrefy at variable rates.

4. Male bodies float in the water with back up, i.e., prone and the female ones with chest up (supine) because of their higher fat contents in the breasts.

SUDDEN DEATH:

Death is said to be sudden or unexpected when a person not known to have been suffering from any disease, injury or poisoning is found death or dies within 24 hours after the onset of terminal illness. Out of all only, 10% of the deaths reported are sudden.

Causes of sudden death;

Sudden death does not mean instantaneous death. A sudden death may be various origins.

Cardiac tamponade;

Cardiac tamponade, as a complication of myocarditis, MI, trauma, etc. can also be the cause of sudden death. Cardiac tamponad is cause of sudden death. Cardiac tamponade is pressure on the heart that occur when blood or fluid builds up in the space between the heart muscle (myocardium) and the outer covering sac of the heart (pericardium).

Chapter 6

ASPHYXIA

ASPHYXIA:

Asphyxia is condition cause by interference with the exchange of oxygen and carbon dioxide in the body.

- Asphyxia literally means defective aeration of blood due to any cause.

ETIOLOGY OF ASPHYXIA:

i. **MECHANICAL / VIOLENT** ; mechanical interference to the passage of air into the respiratory tract by
   - Closure of the external respiratory orifices by closing the nose and the mouth
   - Closure of the air passages by external pressure on the neck or impaction of foreign bodies.
   - Occlusion of the respiratory tract and lungs by fluid.
   - Pressure on the chest in a stampede or collapse of a building.

ii. **PATHOLOGICAL;** Entry of oxygen to the lungs is prevented by disease of the upper respiratory tract or lungs.

iii. **TOXIC OR CHEMICAL;** Cessation of the respiratory movements due to paralysis of the respiratory center in the poisoning with morphine, barbiturates and strychnine. Inhibition of oxidative processes in the tissue preventing the use of oxygen in the blood, e.g. cyanide poisoning.

iv. **ENVIRONMENTAL;** Breathing in vitiated atmosphere as in the high altitude, climbing or flying, or inhalation of CO sewer gas or pure helium.

TRAUMATIC; Blunt trauma to the thorax may result in pneumothorax or heamothorax or pulmonary embolism that will interfere with oxygenation and ventilation by compressing otherwise healthy parenchyma.

v. **POSITIONAL/ POSTURE;** Positional asphyxia is due to peculiar body position that prevents adequate gas exchange.

- In alcoholics or addicts, where the person is unconscious and the upper portion of the body is lower than rest, or neck is forcibly flexed on the chest which prevents normal respiratory movements.
- Positional/restraint asphyxia may occur in hogtying also.

vi. **IATROGENIC;** It is seen during anesthesia.

Clinical effects of asphyxia;

Tardieu's or Bayard's ecchymoses / spots; They are usually round, dark-red, well- defined, pin-head sized supported, e.g. conjunctiva, face, epiglottis, subpleural surface of lungs, heart, meninges and thymus.

- They tend to be better made out in fair skinned persons, readily visible in fresh bodies and disappear with putrefaction.
- It can be seen in other forms of death electrocution, poisoning, coronary thrombosis, in persons on anticoagulants, with bleeding disorders such as scurvy, leukemia and thrombocytopenia, but distribution is more generalized.

Chapter 7

HANGING

HANGING

Hanging or self suspension is the form of asphyxia which is caused by suspension of the body by a ligature which encircles the neck, the constricting force being at least part of the weight of the body.

CLASSIFICATION;

ON THE BASIS OF POSITION OF THE KNOT;

TYPICAL HANGING; when the point of suspension is placed centrally over the occiput. i.e the knot is at the nape on the back.

ATYPICAL HANGING; knot of ligature is anywhere other than on the occiput.

ON THE BASIS OF DEGREE OF SUSPENSION;

COMPLETE HANGING; body is fully suspended and no part of the body touches the ground. Constricting force is weight of the body.

INCOMPLETE OR PARTIAL HANGING;

Lower part of the body is touching the ground or sitting, kneeling, lying down or prone position. Weight of the head acts as the constricting force[1,2,3].

CAUSES OF DEATH;

a) **ASPHYXIA;** Constricting force of ligature causes compressive narrowing of laryngeal and tracheal lumina , leading to asphyxia.

b) **VENOUS CONGESTION;** Jugular veins are blocked by the ligature which results in stoppage of cerebral circulation; occurs if ligature is made up of broad and soft material.

c) **COMBINED ASPHYXIA AND VENOUS CONGESTIO;** Commonest cause.

d) **CEREBRAL ANEMIA;** it occurs when ligature is made of thin cord.

e) **REFLEX VAGAL INHIBITION;** Leading to sudden cardiac arrest.

f) **FRACTURE/ DISLOCATION OF CERVICAL VERTEBRAE**; It is seen in judicial hanging.

DELAYED DEATHS; Are rare which may be due to;

- Aspiration pneumonia
- Edema of lungs, larynx
- Infections
- Infarction of brain
- Hypoxic encephalopathy
- Abscess of brain

SECONDARY EFFECTS;

Hanging in persons who have recovered are;

- Hemiplegia
- Epileptiform convulsions
- Amnesia
- Cervical cellulitis
- Parotitis
- Retropharyngeal abscess[4.]

FATAL PERIOD;

Death is immediate, if cervical vertebrae are fractured or if the heart is inhibited, rapid if cause is asphyxia and least rapid if coma is responsible. Usual period is 3 to 5 min which may extend to 5 to 8 min of suspension leading to death.

Treatment

1. When death occurs slowly the constriction in the neck is released by raising the body by holding it firmly and pushing it up and then loosening or cutting the ligature material from the point the suspension with help of another person.

2. At once the artificial respiration started by sylvestor's method by putting the patient in prone position and lifting up and down the upper extremity and pressing over the back of lower half of chest. Now a days such a patient is put in a ventilator after endotracheal intubation.

3. The tongue is pulled out and mucus is wiped from mouth,pharynx and nostrils. Mechanical suckers may also be used.

4. Oxygen inhalation or, still better oxygen with 50% carbon diaoxide (carbogen) is tried. Some dr prefers NH3 inhalation and cold perfusion to the head.

5. The diffusible stimulants like coramine, cardiazol, caffeine, lobeline, etc., by injection are given.

6. Warm blankets and hot water bottle may be necessary.

7. Correction of mental aberration may be required after the victim recovers from effects of asphyxia.

8. Venesection may be necessary to relieve distention of the right side of the heart and pulmonary circulation to cerebral congestion.

9. The patient should be watched for 12 to 20 hours after respiration has been established, as death may occur from a relapse of the symptoms.

10. The secondary effects of hanging in subjects who have recovered are sometimes hemiplegia, eliptiform convulsion amnesia dementia

bronchitis haemoptysis cervical cellulitis parotitis and retropharyngeal abscess.

POST-MORTEM APPEARRANCE
External signs on neck and body parts

1.neck is found stretched enlongatedandundalymobil in complete suspetionfor a long time .face is usually congested in cases where the vein were very much pressed upon.it would be found swollen and distorted after setting in of decomposition or putrefection.

2. Eyelids are open, eye balls are protruded, lips are livid and pupils are dilated

3. Finger nails are blue .

4. Tongue may protrude out of the mouth.

5. Hands are clenched.

6. Frothy blood stained mucous is seen in the mouth and the nose.

7. streaks of saliva is seen trickling down from the mouth opposite to the site of the knot in cases of atypical hanging and a typical hanging from centre of lower lips down the chins and over chest in straight lines; its presence is the surest sign of ante–mortem hanging. Ligature material presses on the salivary glands and pushes up the root of tongue backwards and saliva remains in the mouth and not swallowed.

8. External genitalia are found congested, swollen with tergid pelvic organs, in males seminal matter may escape through the urethra . Seminal stains may be seen on garments under garments.

In females, there may be discharge of blood stained mucus per vaginum [commonly mistaken as if rape was commited on her earlier]. Faeces and urine also come out owing to the relaxation of sphinctures.

9. Onset of rigor mortis is slow when there is loss of muscle power but in case of death following convulsion it may set in fast.

Post –mortem stains are seen on the lower part of the body [i.e. hands and feet]and above the ligature mark on the neck . if the body is brought down and kept in supine state from state of hanging with in 6 hrs , secondary areas of light colour post-mortem staining is seen over the back of the chest and abdomen .

10. The most characterstic external sign is presence of ligature material and ligature mark on the neck; production of ligature mark depends on:

a. Nature of cord i.e. soft and firm.

b. Tightness of cord.

c. Width of cord.

d. Period of suspension.

e. Weight of subject.

f. Intervention of some material between the skin and ligature material e.g. tuft of scalp hair on back of neck or long and thick beard on front of neck in females and males respectively. Ligature material is removed from the neck by first steadying knot by putting a ligature with tonned thread over it . Then the ligature material is removed from the neck by cutting at a point opposite to the knot after putting two ligatures with tonned thread on the ligatures material diagonally opposite to the knot.[1-5]

Features of ligature mark

❖ The mark is chocolate, brown coloured, furrowed and situated high up in the front of the neck above the thyroid cartilage i.e. more towards the chin [81% cases], very seldom it is below or on the thyroid cartilage.

❖ It is oblique in position, knot being at a higher level.

❖ It does not completely encircle the neck, but leaves a gap due to presence of knot in the ligature material.

❖ Knot is usually situated between the mastoid process and the angle of the mandible in atypical hanging and on uppermost part of back of neckin typical hanging.

❖ The head is tilted towards the opposite of knot. Maximum tension would be exerted at a place directly opposite the knot where mark would be observed. The position of the Knot is indicated by an irregular area the course of uniform mark. The ligature mark may rarely appear to be almost completely circular, and at the lower part of the neck, if a running noose or a slipping knot is used with a thin and stout ligature material.

❖ If the period of suspension is long, the mark becomes deeply grooved or furrowed and is very well defined.

❖ It will be dark reddish brown or chocolate in colour and skin at the site is dry, hard, shiny and feel parchmentised. The parchmentisation is simply due to desiccation of the skin due to the compression of the cuticle by the ligature material.

❖ This is physical process; almost similar situation can be produced even in a dead body within 2-3 hrs after death but antemortem reaction will be absent.

❖ Depending on the nature of ligature material, there may be abrasions in course of the mark. If pressure is exerted for a long period and ligature material is short and stout, capillaries above and below the ligature material develop increased intracapillary tension at ligature site and capillaries may rupture and produce a minimum linear ecchymosis on either side of ligature mark. This is a strong evidence of suspension during life and not seen in postmortem hanging done by accused.

❖ person to stimulate suicidal hanging after killing the subject by some means e.g, head injuriespoisoningetc , or by strangulation by ligature; ligature mark in such situations does not show evidence of vital or antemortem reaction.[1-5]

LYNCHING:

Lynching is a form of homicidal hanging. A suspect, an accused or an enemy is overpowered by several persons, acting jointly and illegally and hung him by means of a rope from a tree or some similar object.

It was prevalent in North America, where it was practiced by whites on Negroes.

JUDICIAL HANGING;

In case of judicial hanging, the ligature is looped around the neck with the knot under the chin, but sub aural knot is also used.

The drop is at least the height of the victim (5-7 feet) and the hanging is complete. The ligature around the neck causes a forceful jerky impact on the neck at the end of the fall, so as to cause fracture of cervical column with stretching or tearing of cervical spinal cord, but not decapitation. In judicial hangings, odontoid process is usually not fractured[1-3].

References:
1. Basu S.C. , Hand Book Of Forensic Medicine and Toxicology, *thirdedition (2007),* Current Distributors, Lenin Saranee, Calcutta.(page 45 to 50).
2. Modi. Jaising. P, Textbook of Medical Jurisprudence And Toxicology, Twenty *First Edition (1997),* N.M. Tripathi Private Limited, Bombay.
3. Parikh C.K., Parikh's textbook of medical jurisprudence forensic medicine and toxicology, *sixth edition (2011),*C.B.S. Publishers and Distributors, Ansari Road, Darya Ganj, New Delhi. (Page no. 3.40,to 3.46)
4. www.wikipedia.com
5. Krishan Vij Textbook of Forensic medicine and Toxicology, 4th Edt.

Chapter 8

STRANGULATION

STRANGULATION

Definition: it is a form of violent asphyxia death caused by constriction of air passage at the neck by means of a ligature or by any means *other than suspension of the body.*

Classification

- **Ligature strangulation:** When ligature material is used to compress the neck.

- **Manual strangulation or throttling**: when human fingers, palms or hands are used to compress the neck.

- **Mugging:** Strangulation caused by holding the neck of the victim in the bend of elbow or knee of the assailant. It is an attack, usually from behind, and may leave no external or internal injury mark. It is also known as chokehold. This hold is not permitted in wrestling, because of its danger.

- **Bansdola:** A bomboo or stick is placed across the back of the neck and another across the front. Both the ends are tied with a rope due to which the victim is squeezed to death. When a foot or knee is placed across the front of throat and pressed while the victim is lying on ground, same condition will follow. If a stick or foot is used, a bruise is seen in the centre, across the trachea corresponding to the width of the object used.

- **Garroting:** strangulation is caused by compression of the neck by a ligature which is quickly tightened by twisting it with a lever (rod, stick or ruler) known as Spanish windlass which results in sudden loss of consciousness and collapse. Garroting as a mode of execution was

153

practiced in Spain, Portugal and Turkey. An iron collar was tightened by a screw for strangulation.

LIGATURE STRANGULATION

Cause of death

- Asphyxia due to elevation of the larynx and tongue closing the airway at pharyngeal level.
- Cerebral anoxia due to venous congestion.
- Vagal inhibition.
- Rarely, fracture dislocation of cervical vertebrae.

GENERAL FINDINGS

i.   Lungs are congested, edematous with numerous subpleural petechial hemorrhages.

ii. Brain is congested with petechiae in white matter.

iii. All other organs are congested.

SUICIDAL STRANGULATION

- Suicide by strangulation is rare. The victims employ various methods of tightening the ligature, but the person can apply a single or double knot before consciousness is lost.
- In suicidal strangulation, signs of venous congestion are very well developed above the ligature and are especially prominent at the root of tongue.
- The ligature should be found in situ; body should not show signs of violence or marks of struggle.

HOMICIDAL STRANGULATION:

Strangulation should be assumed to be homicidal, until the contrary is proved. Many of the victims are women, and frequently, strangulation in them is associated with sexual intercourse.

Homicide is suspected when:

- There are two or more firm knots, each on separate turns of the ligature.
- Abrasions and fingernail marks are seen.
- The clothing of victim is torn or disarranged, indicating that a struggle when removed is loose.
- The ligature when removed is loose.

Sometimes, homicidal strangulation is feigned by an individual to bring a false charge against his enemy. Hysterical women sometimes feign ikt, without any obvious motive.

ACCIDENTAL STRANGULATION

- Accidental strangling may occur in uterus, when the movement of fetus causes the umbilical cord to encircle the neck.
- Children may get entangled in ropes during play or strangled in their cots.
- Persons under the influence of alcohol, epileptics and imbeciles may be strangled either by a tight scarf or collar or necktie.

PSEUDO OR FALSE STRANGULATION GROOVE

- Sometimes, marks are seen on the neck of dead infants or children. Infants have short neck and these marks are produced from folds in the skin due to bending of the head.
- They are also seen in decomposed bodies with tight collars, buttoned shirt bat the neck or a necklace around the neck.

THROTTLING OR MANUAL STRANGULATION

Definition: asphyxia produced by compression of the neck by human hands.

Cause of death

i.   Asphyxia from obstruction of respiration.
ii.   Cerebral anoxia from interference with cerebral circulation.

iii.   Vagal inhibition from pressure on carotid nerve plexus consisting of fibres of vagus, sympathetic and glossopharyngeal nerves. About half of the deaths are due to vagal inhibition.

Pressure must be applied for 2 min or more to cause death.

Chapter 9

SUFFOCATION

SUFFOCATION

Definition: It is a form of asphyxia caused by mechanical obstruction to the passage of air into the respiratory tract by means other than constriction of neck or drowning.

Classification

 i. Smothering

 ii. Choking

 iii. Gagging

 iv. Overlying

 v. Traumatic asphyxia

 vi. Burking

Smothering

Definition: it is a form of asphyxia caused by mechanical occlusion of external air passages, i.e. the nose and mouth by hand, cloth, plastic bag or other material.

Choking

Definition: It is a form of asphyxia caused by an obstruction within the air-passages by a foreign object, like coin, fruit seed, toffees, candies, fish or any other material.

In an epileptic attack, tongue may fall back on to posterior pharyngeal wall causing choking.

The phases of acute fatal airway obstruction are:

 i. Penetration of the object into the airway.

ii.   Obstruction of the airway.

iii.   Failure to expel once the obstruction has occurred.

Mechanism: initially there is stridor, respiratory distress, coughing and ability of victim to speak. This is followed by a rapid, deep inhalation which causes the foreign object to pass further down the airway. Laryngospasm occur followed by vagal stimulation, leading to arrhythmia and apnea and death.

Cause of death

i.   Asphyxia.

ii.   Vagal inhibition.

iii.   Laryngeal spasm.

iv.   Delayed death from pneumonia, lung abscess or bronchiectasis.

Gagging

Definition: Gagging is a form of asphyxia which results from pushing a gag (rolled up cloth or paper balls) into the mouth, sufficiently deep to block the pharynx. It combines the features of smothering and choking.

Initially, the airway may be patent through nose, but collection of saliva, excessive mucosa causes complete obstruction.

Overlaying

- Overlaying or compression suffocation results from compression of the chest, nose and mouth, so as to prevent breathing.

- It is a form of accidental smothering of an infant by a nursing mother, sharing a bed with her child who may roll over during sleep and occlude the air passages.

- Ethanol intoxication or a medical condition can be a factor depressing an arousal response in the older bed-sharer.

Chapter 10

TRAUMATIC ASPHYXIA/CRUSH ASPHYXIA

TRAUMATIC ASPHYXIA/CRUSH ASPHYXIA

Definition: Asphyxia resulting from respiratory arrest due to mechanical fixation of chest, so that the normal movements of chest wall are prevented.

Causes

i.   Due to house collapse, accidentally or in wars/earthquake.

ii.   Stampede by crowd, running in panic, e.g. due to outbreak of fire a cinema hall/public gathering.

iii. Run over by a vehicle or overturned vehicle (especially tractors).

iv.   Collapse of wall inside a mine or trenches (cave-in) in bunkers of sand or grain.

v.   When held between the buffers of two bogies of a train.

vi.   Restraint of suspects by hogtying practiced in some states in US by the police.

Burking

- It is a combination of homicidal smothering and traumatic asphyxia.

- William burke and William hare killed 16 persons during 1927-28 in Scotland and sold their bodies to Dr. Robert Knox for use as specimens in his anatomy classes in Edinburgh Medical School, in what became known as the case of the body snatchers (West Port murders).

Method: A victim was invited to their house and given alcohol. When drunk, he was thrown on the ground and burke would kneel or sit on the chest and close the nose and mouth with his hands, and Hare used to pull him around the room by the feet.[1,2,3,4]

References:

Basu S.C. , Hand Book Of Forensic Medicine and Toxicology, third edition (2007), Current Distributors, Lenin Saranee, Calcutta.(p. 1-3,10).

Mahanta Putul, Modern Textbook of Forensic Medicine And Toxicology (2014), Jaypee Brothers Medical Publishers, Darya Ganj, New Delhi. (P. 8-13, 16,17,20).

Parikh C.K., Parikh's textbook of medical jurisprudence forensic medicine and toxicology, sixth edition (2011),C.B.S. Publishers and Distributors, Ansari Road, Darya Ganj, New Delhi. (P. 1.3, 1.4, 1.9, 1.17, 1.19).

Kumar Avinash, Law Of Evidence, third edition (2011), Singhal Law Publications, Burari, Delhi -84. (Page no. 105-106, 130, 172, 176,177,178,209,216).

Chapter 11

DROWNING

DROWNING

Drowning is the process of experiencing respiratory impairment from submersion/ immersion in liquid.

- Implicit in this definition is that a liquid air interface is present at the entrance to the victim's airway which prevents the individual from breathing oxygen.
- Outcome may include delayed morbidity, delayed or rapic death, or life without morbidity.
- Terms wet or dry drowning, active or passive drowning near-drowning and secondary drowning would be discarded.

CASSIFICATION;

I. TYPICAL OR WET DROWNING;

Water is inhaled into the lungs and the victim has severe chest pain. It is also known as primary drowning.

II. ATYPICAL DROWNING; or dry drowning

DRY DROWNING;

- ❖ In dry drowning, water does not enter the lungs due to laryngeal spasm induced by small amounts of water entering the larynx.
- ❖ Seen in 1 to 2 % of cases.
- ❖ Death may be extremely rapid and time elapsed is insufficient for typical drowning to occur.

ASPHYXIAL DEATHS

Asphyxial literally means 'pulselessness'.

Asphyxial is a very broad term relating to the 'inadequate aeration of blood'. Thus, there is hypoxia (lack of oxygen) and hypercapnia (excess of carbon dioxide). The brain, being the most sensitive to lack of oxygen's, is the earliest to suffer in all types of asphyia.

Barcroft (1920) postulated that anoxia (absence of oxygen) in the blood is possible in three ways, namely anoxic, anemic and stagnant anoxia. Peters and slyke (1931) added a fourth group and called it histotoxic anoxia.

Chapter 12

STARVATION DEATH

STARVATION DEATH

Definition;

By definition, starvation is the process that may occur from the long and continuous deprivation of food needed to maintain the normal health. It can also be defined as an act of depriving the food or subjecting to famine.

Malnutrition is a state of poor nutrition, which can result from insufficient or absorb foods.

Cachexia is general lack of nutrition and wasting occurring in the course of a chronic debilitating disease. Emaciation means loss of body weight.

By depriving the body of nutrition, starvation slowly allows the body to consume its own reverves, including muscle, fat and organs, up to the point of complete system shutdown and death.

Types of starvation;

Starvation is usually of two types;

Acute starvation

Chronic starvation.

Acute starvation;

This condition results from sudden and complete cessation of food and water.

Chronic starvation;

This condition results from gradual deficiency in the supply of food and water.[1,2,3,4]

Fatal period;

If both water and food are completely withdrawn, death occurs in 10 to 12 days.[1, 3.]

If food alone is withdrawn, death usually occurs when about 70% to 90% of the body fat and 20% of the body proteins are lost. Newborns may survive for 7 to 10 days without food or water.[2, 3]

FACTORS INFLUENCING THE FATAL PERIOD;

Age: the young adult suffer from deprivation worse than old, as the old person have an low requirement. Adults bear starvation better than the children do.

Sex: female withstands starvation for a longer period because of higher storage of fat in the body.

Nutritional status of body; fatty, healthy people bear it better than ill and thin.

Temperature; exposure o extreme of temperature hastens the death.

Physical exertion; an active physical activity hurries death.

Clinical features;

Acute starvation:

The person becomes hungry for the first 30-48 hours, followed by stomachache, which is relieved by pressure.

Features after 4 to 5 days of starvation;

- General emaciation, absorption of the subcutaneous fat , eyes are sunken and glistening; mydriasis; hollowed checks with visible bony prominences.
- Dry and cracked lips, coated tongue wit intolerable thirst.
- Thick and scanty saliva with weak and whispering voice.
- Dry, rough and inelastic skin, this may be wrinkled and pigmented.

- Thin abdominal concave and limbs, with loss of muscular power with progressive muscular weakness that may be severe in due course of time.
- Cardiovascular changes; slow pulse at rest, paroxysmal tachycardia on exertion. The temperature is subnormal.
- Constipation is common, but diarrhea. And dysentery may supervene towards the end of life.
- Scanty, turbid and highly concentrated urine, with evidence of acidosis.
- Constant weight loss is most marked.
- At the last stage, body is reduced to an extreme state of emaciation characterized by prominent ribs, with concavities in the intercostals spaces and sunken supraclavicular fossae.
- Intellect remains clear though in some cases, delusions and hallucinations of slight and hearing occur.

Chronic starvation;

The changes following chronic starvation are constant and develop in a constant order as follows;

- Loss of well-being, hunger and the easy fatigability.
- Mental and physical lethargy and easy fatigability
- Progressive loss of weight, which is rapid in the first 6 months
- Increasing cachexia, the body weight is reduced by about 40% of the normal
- Pigmentation and development of anemia.
- Hypothermia, peripheral vascular stasis in the cold and hypotension.
- Edema, first in the feet then other parts of the lower limbs.
- Reduced resistance to infection causes diarrhea, dysentery, tuberculosis, etc.
- Lowered blood sugar, proteins, chlorides and cholesterol. NPN and urea are raised
- In females, irregular menstruation can occur.

Causes of starvation[1-5];

The main cause of starvation is an imbalance between energy intake and energy spending. This imbalance can arise from some medical conditions and/or circumstantial situations.

Circulatory failure due to brown atrophy of the heart or recurrent infection.

- Dehydration
- Hypothermia
- Electrolyte imbalance, etc.
- Postmortem findings
- External examination;

Body is emaciated, characterized by prominent ribs, with concavities in the intercostals space and sunken supraclavicular fossae.

Rigor mortis sets in and disappears early. Pale face, inelastic and pigmented skin, absorption of the subcutaneous fat, sunken eyes; mydriasis; hollowed sheeks with visible bony prominences.

- Dry and cracked lips, coated tongue.
- Dry, rough with inelastic skin, this may be wrinkled and pigmented.

Atrophied and darker muscles due to increase in lip chrome. Thin abdominal concave and limbs. Edemas are seen around the ankles and inside the thighs. In wet type, there is edema of the face, trunk and limbs with ascites and pleural effusions.

- Dry hair, lustreless with brittle nails.
- Children's skeleton shows spinal curvature, rickets and dental defects. Osteomyelitic changes are seen in adult.
- Body looks pale due to reduced blood volume and marked anemia.
- Internal examination;

- Fat is nearly absent in the subcutaneous tissues and also in the omentum, mesentery and in the internal organs, but the fat around the female breast and the orbit is persistent till last moment.

- Subepicardial fat becomes replaced by a watery gelatinous material.

- Stress fractures may occur.

- All organs and tissues are pale and show changes of premature senility.

- General reduction in size and weight of all the organs except the brain, which is sometimes pale and soft.

- Heart is smaller due to brown atrophy with empty chambers.

- Lungs are pale, collapsed and exude very little blood on cut section. There may be edema and hypostatic basal congestion.

- Stomach and intestines shows atrophied mucosa stained with bile.

- Intestinal walls appear like tissue paper with atrophied mucosa.

- Bowel contains offensive watery fluid and gas.

References:

1. Basu S.C. , Hand Book Of Forensic Medicine and Toxicology, third edition (2007), Current Distributors, Lenin Saranee, Calcutta.(p 3-10).
2. Mahanta Putul, Modern Textbook of Forensic Medicine And Toxicology (2014), Jaypee Brothers Medical Publishers, Darya Ganj, New Delhi. (P 8-13,16-17,20).
3. Parikh C.K., Parikh's textbook of medical jurisprudence forensic medicine and toxicology, sixth edition (2011),C.B.S. Publishers and Distributors, Ansari Road, Darya Ganj, New Delhi. (P1.3, 1.4, 1.9, 1.17, 1.19).
4. Kumar Avinash, Law Of Evidence, third edition (2011), Singhal Law Publications, Burari, Delhi -84. (Page no. 105-106, 130, 172, 176-178, 209, 216).
5. Modi. Jaising. P, Textbook of Medical Jurisprudence And Toxicology, Twenty First Edition (1997), N.M. Tripathi Private Limited, Bombay.

Chapter 13

HUMAN RIGHTS, CUSTODIAL TORTURE AND DEATHS

HUMAN RIGHTS, CUSTODIAL TORTURE AND DEATHS;

"You can change me you can torture me, you can ever destroy this body, but you can never imprison my mind". (**Mahatma Gandhi**).

TORTURE

TORTURE CAN BE SIMPLY DESCRIBED; as the act to inflict intense physical, psychological, emotional pain in order to punish, coerce or afford sadistic pleasures. According to 1984 United Nations Convention Against Torture, it is defined as ' any act by which severe pain or suffering, whether physical or mental, is intentionally inflicted on a person for such purposes as obtaining from him or a third person information or a confession, punishing him for an act he or a third person has committed or is suspected of having committed, or intimidating or coercing him or a third person, or for any reason based on discrimination of any kind, when such pain or suffering in inflicted by or at the instigation of or with the consent or acquiescence of a public official or other person acting in an official capacity. It does not include pain or suffering arising only from, inherent in or incidental to, lawful sanction.

Laws against torture;

The UNDHR had a wider role to safeguard various aspecs of human rights, in general and torture. Specific International treaties were passed with the passage of time.

Each state party shall take effective legislative, administrative, judicial or other measures to prevent acts of torture in any territory under its jurisdiction.

No exceptional circumstances whatsoever, whether a state of war or a threat or war, internal political instability is any other public emergency, may be invoked as a justification of torture.

An order from a superior officer or a public authority may not be invoked as a justification of torture.

No state party shall expel, return or extradite a person to another state where there is substantial ground for believing the he would be in danger of being subjected to torture.

Purpose o torture;

- Broadly, use of torture was justified for following reasons;
- To solve crimes as a tool of interrogation
- To maintain social control
- To defend the ruling state from internal and external threats
- To force confessions
- Ethnic cleansing
- Extortion
- Types of torture;
- Physical torture
- Sexual torture
- Psychological torture
- Pharmacological torture

Chapter 14

ANESTHETIC PROCEDURES AND DEATH

ANESTHETIC PROCEDURES AND DEATH;

Since introduction of anesthetic agents in facilitating surgical procedures, it has been established as about. But occasionally, it has turned out to be bane for treating doctors and even patient. Biomedical researchers have shown a reasonable concern in preventing and treating preoperative complications, whether surgical or anesthetic in nature or origin.

Such decline have been attributed to introduction of better monitoring devices, (i.e. multipara monitor- displaying indicators like pulse oxymetry , blood pressure,SpO_2, ECG, and $EtCO_2$) of course coupled with better training of operative team members. Howevers to screen out 'exclusive anesthetic death' among perioperative events may have many inherent limitations.

Classification of anesthetic deaths:

Gordon and Shapiro classified the anesthetic death into two broad groups. During the administration of anesthesia but not related to anesthesia. Death which are direct result of administration of anesthesia

TYPES OF ANESTHESIA USED IN SURGICAL PROCEDURE

PREANESTHETIC MEDICATION

- Pentazocine (fortwin)- opioid
- Butorphenol-opioid
- Tramadol-synthetic opioids
- Midazolam-benzodiazepine
- Dynapar- NSAIDs

Mechanism of action;

Anesthetic agent potentiates the action of inhibitory transmitter GABA to open CL-channels. Whatever may be the pathway, common adverse effects are either respiratory or cardiac in origin in the form of depression or dysfunction. The common agent and their side effects.

Causes of death due to general anesthesia;

- Over dose of anesthetic agent.
- Anesthesia to wrong patients.
- Wrong connection to gas machine, which may cause unexpected mixture of dangerous gases.
- Death due to hypoxia due to respiratory depression, hypoventilation, excessive muscle relaxation, laryngeal spasm due to inhalation of vomitus, etc.
- Precipiation of myocadial ischemia because fuse of IV Pentothal which is depressing to heart.
- Wrong posture of the body leads to paralysis of a limb or its part.
- Faulty anesthetic equipment.
- Failure to diagnose the impending danger during monitoring of the vital sign
- Unknown etiology. [1,2,3]

References:

1. Basu S.C. , Hand Book Of Forensic Medicine and Toxicology, third edition (2007), Current Distributors, Lenin Saranee, Calcutta.
2. Mahanta Putul, Modern Textbook of Forensic Medicine And Toxicology (2014), Jaypee Brothers Medical Publishers, Darya Ganj, New Delhi.
3. Parikh C.K., Parikh's textbook of medical jurisprudence forensic medicine and toxicology, sixth edition (2011),C.B.S. Publishers and Distributors, Ansari Road, Darya Ganj, New Delhi.

Chapter 15

INJURY AND WOUND

INJURY AND WOUND

Injury as defined in section 44 of IPC mean any harm or damage illegally caused to one body , mind , reputation and property by another human being,[1]"

A **wound** is a type of injury in which skin is torn, cut, or punctured (an *open* wound), or where blunt force **trauma** causes a **contusion** (a *closed* wound) or damages the **dermis** of the skin.[1]

Medico legal classification of injuries

According to nature of injury to body

Mechanical Injuries

1) Abrasion

2) Bruise

3) Wounds

- ❖ incised
- ❖ Lacerated
- ❖ Stabs
- ❖ Gunshot
- ❖ Injury to internal organs or structures with or without any external lesion.

Some important weapons cause mechanical injuries

1) Hard ,blunt or rough weapons
2) Sharp cutting weapons
3) Fire arm
   Long barreled and short barreled
4) Bomb blast

Thermal Injuries

1) Burn and scalds
2) Injuries caused by electricity lighting x ray and other radio active substances

Chemical Injuries

1) Corrosive acids
2) Corrosive alkalies[1]

According to severity of injury

1) Simple
2) Dangrous
3) Grievous

1) Simple wound

Though a pin prick can cause death by causing vagal Shock leading to cardiac arrest, the term simple wound may be used by doctor to signify that these wound commonly occur in day to day life and heal rapidly within one or two weeks and without incapacitating a person from his daily for more that two week.[1]

2) Dangerous wound

These wound are large in size and more sever in nature than simple wound generally they are often fatal wounds. There is always an apprehension or danger to life. This fact should be at once intimated to the local magistrate through local police station and arrangements are to made for recording of dying declaration .danger to life should be considered imminent I in compound fracture of the **skull wound** involving a large artery, vital internal structure rupture of internal organ ,etc. injuries which prove fetal by causing intercurrent infection or complication like tetnus, gas gangrene etc are not considered as immediately dangerous .but accused person would not get any defense or benefit for the death precipitated by infections of the wound which resulted from the criminal intention and act responsible for primary injury.[2]

3) Grievous hurt

It is a special type of dangerous wound. These are the injuries or bodily pain which is commonly cause the suffers to have either permanent damage or loss of a part of the body or incapacitates him from doing his normal work for more than

20 days. It may be mentioned that all dangerous wounds may also be griavous in nature but all griavous hurts may not be dangerous wounds.[1]

Conditions

1. Emasculation-Injuries to the testis, deprivation of masculinity of a person by castration or cutting off the male organ, injuries to the spinal cord involving sex centres at the lumber segment is also important, as it may cause impotency
2. Permanent privation of sight of one or both eyes
3. Permanent privation of hearing of one or both ears
4. Permanent privation of any membrane or joint
5. Permanent disfigurement of head and face
6. Fruture of a bone[2']

According to Body Parts Involved

1) Head injury
2) Spinal injury[1'']
3) Thoraco-abdominal injuries
4) Limb injuries

According to the Nature of the Object Causing the Injury

1) By hard rough object
2) By soft malleable object
3) By sharp objects
4) By pointed objects, sharp, or blunt
5) By guns[1]

ABRASION

This is caused by a rubbing of the cuticle or superficial layers of the skin by some rough or hard substance by finger nails or bite by teeth. They are caused by a very slight violence and may be associated with or without bruise. A blow with a hard and blunt substance on an yielding parts like anterior abdominal wall, may not cause an abrasion there. Multiple extensive abrasions with severe injuries on different parts of the associated with black marks of grease, dirt, mud, etc indicate street or traffic accident .Tags of epithelium and furrows indicate the direction of force[.1,2]

TYPES

1. Scratch: caused by pointed object passing across the skin eg. Nail, thorn, pin etc

2. Graze: caused by movement of hard rough object in contact with skin eg. Glancing kick with boot, road traffic accidents.[3]

3. Pressure abrasion

4. Impact abrasion[1-5]

DIFFERECE BETWEEN ANTE-MORTUM AND POST-MORTUM ABRATION

ANTE MORTUM	POST MORTUM
Surface is moist due to exudation of serum and may show sing of bleeding	Surface is dry because there is no exudation of serum.
Formation of raddish brown scap	No scab is found
No parchmentisation of skin under the abraded area.	Parchmentisation of the exposed area.

AGE OF ABRASION

- ❖ Birth red with oozing of serum
- ❖ 24 hours bright red scab
- ❖ 2-3 days reddish brown scab
- ❖ 4-6 days epithelium grows and covers the defects under the scap
- ❖ By 7th day-scab falls, leading to depigmented area
- ❖ By 14th day completely normal skin[2,3]

Medicolegal Importance of Abrasion

- ❖ Abrasion may be only external indication of serious internal damage. Abrasion over neck indicates hanging or substance or strangulation.
- ❖ Abrasion over inner aspects of thigh, genitalia, breast, and lower abdomen may indicate sexual assault.
- ❖ Extensive abrasion all over the body may be seen in road accidents.

- Over lips, mouth and nostrils abrasion may indicate suffocation.
- Elliptical abrasion cased by teeth bites or abrasion caused finger nails indicate struggle in self defence.
- Imprint abrasions like bumper or grill marks, tyre-tread mark.
- Age of abrasion may indicate age of assault or incidence[1]"

BRUISE

It is a type of mechanical injury characterized by patch of discoloration caused by extravasation of blood in tissues, due to rupture of blood vessels, commonly capillaries as a result of application of blunt force trauma .In this wound, and there is no solution of continuity of the skin.

Cause

The violence is caused by the fist, blow or kick or by any hard and blunt weapons such as stick, brick and stone and also by fall, crush, etc. The injured area becomes dark reddish to blue in colour and its surface may or may not show any abrasion. There are always some pain and swelling which are due to the rupture and crushing of the underlying tissues and the blood vessels , producing an etravasasation or effusion of blood into the tissues, The swelling is also due to the presence of cellular exudates.[3]"

When a bruise is associated with pain and swelling it is called ecchymosis. In ecchymosis, there is a diffuse extravasation of blood over a wider area under the seat of violence .large size extravasation of blood are commonly called contusion.

SUPERFICIAL BRUISE

It generally appears at the seat of violence within a short time– a few minutes to one hour after the injury .It is bluish red in colour. But it may appear in much shorter time, if skin involved is thin and the underlying tissue is lax, as in eyelids and scrotum.[4]"

DEEP BRUISE

It takes a longer time–two, three or several days after the injury to makes its appearance on surface and frequently, the extraverted blood gravitates in the tissues and makes its appearance at a site, which is at a considerable distance from the actual seat of violence e.g

- ❖ A blow on forehead or a fall on vertex may produce black eyes
- ❖ A blow or kick in calf region of leg may cause a bruise round about the ankle.[4]

Site and Extent of Bruise Generally Depend Upon

- ❖ Looseness of subcutaneous tissues
- ❖ Vascularity of the part
- ❖ Condition of the blood clotting mechanism of an individual–in scurvy, haemophilia and purpura
- ❖ Severity of the blow
- ❖ Condition of the blood vessels–arteriosclerosis [4"]

Shape

Shape of the bruise may depend on the shape of the weapon used- irregular in an irregular stone, elongated or cylindrical in lathi, or round when the striking surface of hammer is used. In a bruise due to strick by cane, there will be linear depressed area separating two raised parallel bruises. The gap in between two bruise marks indicates the diameter of the cane. The central parts is depressed apparently, as both sides are raised due to the increased intracapillary tension. In the depressed area the capillaries are compressed by the cane and in the raised areas, the extra blood is pushed from these compressed capillaries leading to increased intra capillary tension on either side of the area struck by cane. Hence, these capillaries rupture giving raise to two bruise .on palm of hand and soles of feet cane produce single line bruise. A bruise may be accompanied by laceration of the subjacent tissue, future of an underlying bone or rupture of an internal organ. There may be rupture of internal organ without the presence of the superficial bruise on the abdominal wall. Bruise regarded as simple wound[5,6"]

The time, when the bruise has made its appearance, may be determined by the change in colour of the extravasted blood owing to the alteration in blood pigment[.1"]

AGE OF BRUISE

- ❖ Just after infliction it is red the colour changes start in the peripheral portion and consist a gradual passing from violet to blue on 2nd to 3rd day(reduction of haemoglobin)
- ❖ It become brown on the 5th day and green by the 7t to 14th days. Bruise ordinarily heal by 2 weeks

- After this period, skin assumes its normal colour .This period is not always constant, it may vary from 5- 15 days in superficial bruise. A bruise disappears rapidly in healthy well nourished adults and slowing in old persons.
- Deep seated ecchymosis may not show any such colour changes for long time, eg; cerebral contusion.[5"]

MEDICOLEGAL QUESTIONS

Whether the bruise is accidental, homicidal, suicidal or artificially produced ?

Accidental Bruise: May be caused on different parts of the body in the street accidents or in fall from a height and may be associated with other injuries.

Homicidal Bruise: Position, shape, size, number and arrangement of bruises may help in determining this. It may be present on any part of the body.

Suicidal Bruise: May happen when a person jumps from a height or due to blunt objects.

Artificial Bruise: Bruises like areas may be produced artificially by the application of vegetable irritants like chitra. Lachitra, Marking nuts, or dhobi nuts (semicarpus anacardium). When juices of these articles are applied over the body, it produces a stain, which is very much similar to a bruise.[6"]

INCISED WOUNDS

It is produced by sharp cutting instruments, such as knife, razor safety razor blades swords dagger chopper i.e by objects which have sharp cutting edges. It can be caused by three ways.[7"]

i. Striking, **ii.** Drawing and **iii.** sawing.

Characters

- Its edges are regular, clean-cut retracted and everted, except in neck and scrotum, where edges are inverted owing to the conraction of underlying platysma and dartos tunica respectively, attached to skin of those regions
- It is somewhat spindle shaped with maximum widening at the central part.
- Lengths is the greatest of three dimensions i.e length is greater than the breath and the depth
- Breath is usually greater than the thickness of the cutting blade

- The gapping is greater if the underlying muscles are dividing across or cut obliquely
- Hemorrhage is excessive on account of the clear division of blood vessels. So long the heart is beating; there will be sprouting of arterial blood from the cut end of the artery.
- The edges of wound may appear to be irregular in cases where skin in loose, ie., in the neck and scrotum ,owing to a fold of skin being rolled up or puckered in front of the weapon ,before the skin is dividing.[4"]

Weapons used

From the nature of the incised wound, the type of cutting weapon may be guessed.

1. Light ones, such as razor, knife etc, produce incised wound by striking, drawing or by sawing.[4"]

- Drawing cuts are usually deeper at start, gradually become shallow, till at the end only skin is cut, often terminating in mere scratch, called tailing. The tail indicates the end parts and therefore the relatives position of the accused and the victim can be judged in homicidal cases, or in suicidal cases one can say which hand been used .
- Sawing cuts have more than one cut due to see-saw movement at the beginning, but only one at the other end.
- Beveling cuts occurs, when the weapon is applied over the body in an oblique or tangential way [in pairing of pencil or cutting by daos]

2. Heavy weapons [swords, axes, choppers, daos, etc] when hit vertically produce chop wounds of greater severity than light ones.They are usually homicidal .but may be suicidal as lunatic

3. Incised wound, made by curved weapons like dao, sickle or tangi will make a single wound, when applied over the convex portions of the body.[3"]

Medicolegal Importance

Incised wounds may be suicidal, homicidal, accidental and self inflicted.

- Homicidal cases may occur in any part of the body, commonly on the neck, head and trunk. They may also be found on the inner side of forearm or hand of the victim in his attempt to ward off the attempt.

- ❖ Suicidal wound found in the accessible parts only are usually caused by light weapons. Commonly they are on the throat .The indicates which hand has been used.
- ❖ Accidental wound may be on any parts of the body, commonly on the hand and the fingers during handling of knife, razor, safety razor, blades.
- ❖ Self inflicted wounds are always slight in nature and in accessible parts of the body. They are more or less parallel to each other. These are produce on ones own body to bring a false charge against another person.

Defence Wounds. Defence wound result from the immediate and instinctive reaction of the victim to save himself.[1]

LACERATED WOUNDS

They are the results of splitting, tearing, stretching, or crushing of tissues and are generally caused by the heavy weights, hard and blunt instruments, fali on some hard object , teeth and nails or machinery , railway or traffic accidents as well as by claws or horn of wild animals. It is more a tearing than cutting of tissues because of blunt force hitting the body surface.

Characters

- ❖ The margins of the wound are irregular, ragged and inverted.
- ❖ The tissues are torn and not cut. Deeper tissues are unevenly divided with tags of tissues showing in the wound cavity.
- ❖ The adjacent parts may be divided abraded or contused.
- ❖ There is infiltration of blood inside the tissues.
- ❖ Bleeding will not be marked, owing to crushing of the blood vessels. Blood vessels are torn across irregularly and not cut cleanly as in incised wound; haemorrhage is less than in an incised wound.
- ❖ Chance of infection by tetanus, gas gangrene or pyogenic organism is much more. Lacerated wound are usually not so dangerous unless accompanied by other deep seated lesions like fractures of the bone and injury to vital internal organs.[1-7]

INCISED LOOKING LACERATED WOUNDS

Whenever the skin is stretched ,over a bone or over a sharp ridge of bone, e.g. scalp, face, orbital margin, chin, shin of tibia or external genital organs of a female subject, any hurt with hard and blunt weapon or a fist ,blow or a kick over these parts may produce a lacerated wound, which looks like an incised wound.

Such a wound is always produced by hard and blunt weapon. On examination with a magnifying glass, the margins of wound will appear irregular, ragged and inervated and there is certain degree of bruising or contusions of the adjacent tissues .The hairs of the scalp will be found presented into the wound cavity and hair fibres are crushed. The lacerations are so minute that they are not ordinarily visible to naked eye.[4]

Medicolegal aspect

It may be homicidal, suicidal or accidental.

Homicidal: It occurs in any parts of the body and are produced by blows with hard and blunt weapons.

Suicidal: These is very rare and **accidental** it occurs any parts of the body in street accident.[1]

DIFFERENCE BETWEEN SUICIDAL AND HOMICIDAL WOUNDS[1]

POINT	SUICIDAL	HOMICIDAL
POSITION	ACCESSIBLE PARTS ONLY	NO FIXED SITE
NATURE OF WOUNDS	USUALLY INCISED AND GUN SHOOT WOUND	LACERATED WOUND
SEVERITY	MOSTLY SUPER FACIAL	MOSTLY SEVERE

STAB WOUNDS OR PUNCHURED WOUNDS

They are commonly produced by the pointed tip of sharp object or instrument being driven through the skin as opposed to its cutting edge being applied over the skin. Generally they are caused by the sharp edged pointed piercing and stabbing weapons such as knifes dagger bayonet arrow etc. The similar type of wound may be caused by a fall on pointed projection like railings or by horns of wild animals .The edges of such instruments are commonly blunt.

When the edges of the weapon are sharp, the wound produced is an incised, punctured, perforating and penetrating wound. When they are blunt, it produces a lacerated, punctured perforating and penetrating wound.

In this situation when depth of the wound is greater of three dimensions it is called punctured wound. When a printed end of a weapon enters into a natural body cavity such as thoracic, abdominal, joint cavities or tunica vaginalis in the scortum, it is called a penetrating wound when the wound pierces the body parts through and through, it is known as perforating wound.

Characters

- ❖ Depth of the wound is the greatest of all three dimensions. The depth of the wound is produced by the length of the cutting blade of weapon introduced and its length and breath produced by the breath thickness of the cutting blade of weapon respectively .The wound may be greater in depth than the length of weapons n the yielding parts lik anterior abdominal wall due to the pressure exerted at the site of the stabbing.

- ❖ Breath of the stab wound may be less than that of the weapons used as the skin and the subcutaneous tissues contract on withdrawal of the weapon.

- ❖ Edges are retracted cleanly cut or lacerated according to the nature of instrument used.In wounds produced by sharp cutting weapons like knives ,dagger ,beyonets or by similar instruments, surface wound will be an incised one, whereas with a pick axe or with horns of animals which have blunt edges, the margins will be found to be irregular bruised and lacerated.[1,2']

- ❖ There may not be any stain of blood on the withdraw weapon blood having been wiped off by garments cloth.

- ❖ Surface wound may larger than the actual breath of weapon due to its withdrawal by drawing along a slightly different direction resulting in the enlargement of wound.

- ❖ One punctured wound may have more than one track in side if the weapon is withdrawn partially diverted to another direction and then reintroduce the same weapon stabbed in different direction will produce different length of the wounds.

This stabbing weapon may have a single or double cutting edge from the shape of the surface wound the character of the weapon can be judged in single cutting edge example pencile knife one side is acute angle and other slightly curved example wedge shaped while in a double cutting edge example dagger the surface wound form spindle shape.

There are some degger which have got projection on blunt edge or surface wound will show four angles.

Punctured wounds are sometimes found in situation like axilla inner canthus. Nape of neck, groin, rectum, and vagina these are not easily detected and are called concealed punctured wounds the brain is injured by stabbing through fourth ventricle a common technique four infanticide. Great care should be taken in probing the depth of a punctured wound. This may be done by a blunt probe or by a rubber catheter in an operation theatre.

Perforating wounds have entrance and exist with a tract in between.

Margins will be clean out or ragged according to the nature of weapon used. But, it will be inverted at the site of entrance and everted at the site of exist, provided the wound is in situ. But the weapon is withdrawn after inflicting the character may be reversed.[1-6]

Dagger wound is bigger at the entrance and the smaller at the exist. While a gunshot wound is smaller at the entrance, but wider at the exist.

Danger of stab wounds

- ❖ Shock
- ❖ Haemorrhage
- ❖ Injury to vital organs

Medicolegal aspects

Stab wound may suicidal, homicidal, and accidental.

Suicidal; usually situated at the throat, cardiac area

Homicidal; they are on nay part of the body[5]

DIFFERENCE BETWEEN INCISED LACERATED AND PUNCTURED WOUND[1]

Points	Incised wound	Lacerated wound	Punctured wound
Site	Anywhere	Bony prominence	Chest or abdomen

Shape	Linear	irregular	Linear or irregular
Abrasion on edges	Absent except in chops	present	absent
Haemorrhage	Profuse and external	Slight and external	Acc. To site and internal

GUN SHOOT WOUND

These are caused by projectiles discharged from firearms by firing of a cartridge and show the characteristic of lacerated wound, but the character varies acc. to the **Nature of the projectile: shot or pellets and bullet.**

- ❖ Velocity of the projectile at the moment of impact.
- ❖ Distance of the firearm from the body at the time of discharge
- ❖ Angle of impact: firearm basically consists of a metallic tube known as barrel. Inside diameter of barrel is known as bore. The bore is smooth in shot gun, the bore is longitudinal grooved which are also twisting spirally. In case of pistols , machines guns , ak47 and they discharge bullet

The barrel of the gun has two ends

- ❖ Open and distal end known as muzzle
- ❖ Closed end known as breech end

At the breeched end lies the special structure called the MAGAZINE which houses or contains cartridges just below the magazine or behind the magazine and in front of the magazine lies another special C shaped structure with concavity forwards called TRIGGER this is usually kept locked by mean of a safety catch. When the safety catch is released and the trigger is voluntarily pulled backward by the index finger a firing pin strikes the center of the base of the cartridge case. When there is detonation of percussion cup contents and ignition of propellant charge powder with formation of high volume of gases, the expansive force of which propel out the projectile along with flame, hot gases, black smoke and unburnt propellant charge powder particles. The diameter of the bore is expressed by numbers, eg: 12,16,18, in case of smooth bore guns and decimal of inches in case of rifled firearms{eg:22, 303, in case of rifles, AK47 and 32, and 45 in case of revolvers and pistols].

What is a 12 bore gun?

It indicates the number of lead balls of equal shape size and weight and each ball fitting snugly and tightly in the bore of the gun [smooth bore]

Characteristics

These are nothing but special type lacerated, punctured, perforating and penetrating wounds.

1. They generally produce two wounds or opertures one at the entrance and at the exist of the projectile.

2. Wounds is very erratic and circuitous in its course due to the peculiar course of the bullet in the body.

Wound of entrance

- ❖ Smaller than the diameter of projectile due to the elasticity of the skin
- ❖ Rounded, when projectile strikes the body at right and oval , when it strikes obliquely.
- ❖ Edges of the wound: inverted and ecchymosed.They may be everted in:
- (a) Fatty persons due to protrusion of fat into the wound and in decomposed bodies from the expansile action of gases of putrefection.
- (b) Wadding, pieces of clothing or other debris may be found lodged in the wound.
- (c) Surrounding skin will be scorched and tattooed with particles of unconsumed powder, if the firearm is discharged at a close range.[1,2,7]

Wound of exit

It is commonly caused by bullets and not by pellets. It may be ragged and torn, if the projectile is discharged at close quarters or has passed through the bone or in deformed after striking elsewhere.[1]

These characteristics of the wound are due to the wobble of the projectile; eversion of the margin is seen. Fragments of bone expelled from the body with the projectile or the splinter pieces of the projectile produce it. The wound of exit is generally larger than the wound of entrance.

FACTORS MODIFYING APPEARANCE OF GUNSHOT WOUNDS

Natural of projectiles

Bullets are discharged by rifled firearm and pellets [shots of different size] come out of smooth bore firearm {shotgun}. **Following are the features:**

- ❖ Large bullets cause greater damage.
- ❖ Round bullets cause larger wound, conical bullets cause extensive lacerations.
- ❖ Modern high velocity bullet are like elongated cones and for greater velocity, thcy may pass straight and direct through the body without any deflection or deviation .In these cases of wound entry and exist are both round and similar in appearance without much brusising or laceration of the surrounding parts.
- ❖ Gun power, wards and pellets [shot] sometime produce frightful laceration of the internal organ[1,4,3]

Velocity of projectile

High velocity bullets show following characteristics:

- ❖ Clean, circular, punched out aperture or slit like that of a stabbing wound.
- ❖ Not deflected, even if it strikes a bone in its way but may cause comminution or splintering of the bone.

DISTANCE BETWEEN FIREARM AND THE TARGET

Flam: travel for 3" to4"{8 to 10} and produce singeing of hair and epidermal burn of skin surrounding wound of entrance.

Hot gases and smoke: travel for 6" to 8" and produce blackening and epidermal burn of skin around wound of entrance.

Unburnt propellant charge powder: travel for 24"to 30" and produce tattooing around wound of entrance.

VARIOUS FIREARM WOUND

(i). Shot Gun Wounds

Close to or a few cm of the body

Shot enters in the one mass like a single bullet up to 1 meter. A large irregular wound contused edges is produced. The wad and the gases produce great lacerations and rupture of the deeper tissues. Particle of unburnt powder are driven to some distance through the wound.[2"]

(ii). Rifel Wound

The wound inflicted on the body are similar to pistol wounds, but produce more damage.

(iii). Contact Wound

The burning and tattooing is not much and may be absent.

(iv). Skull Wound

In the skull wound of entrance shows a punched in hole in the outer table ,while opening on the inner table is large and show beveling .piece of bone from wound of entrance are often drive into the cranial cavity and may establish the bullet track.[1,7]

Rrefrence

1. Basu S.C."Foresic medicine and toxicology" current distibutor commercial point 2007.
2. Gupta A.K.Forensic Medicine
3. Mahanta Putul, Modern Textbook of Forensic Medicine and Toxicology 2014, Jaypee Brother Medical Publishers, Darya Ganj, New Delhi
4. Parikh C.K, Parikhs Textbook of Medical Jurisprudence Forensic Medicine and Toxicology Sixth Edition 2011. C.B.S Publishers and Distributors Ansari Road Darya Ganj, New Delhi
5. Kumar Avinash, Law of Evidence 3rd edition 2011 Singhal Law Publisher, Burari Delhi
6. Modi. Jaising Textbook of Medicine of Toxicology Twenty First Edition [1997] N.M Tripathi Private Limited, Bombay
7. Www.Wikipedia.Com

Chapter 16

BURNS AND SCALDS

BURNS AND SCALDS

Definition

Burns are injuries produced by the application of dry heat such as flame, radiant heat or some heated solid substances like metal or glass to the surface of the body.

Injuries caused by friction, lightening, electricity, ultraviolet or infra red light rays, x-rays & corrosive chemical substances are all classified as burns for medico legal purposes.

CLASSIFICATION OF BURNS

Dupuytren has classified burns into the following six degrees according to the nature of their severity.

Modern classification is into three degrees. Only by grouping the first & second (Epidermal) third & fourth (Dermo-epidermal) and fifth & sixth (Deep) degrees together-

EPIDERMAL

First degree- This consist of erythema or simple redness of the skin caused by the momentary application of flame or hot solids or liquids much below the boiling point. It can also produced by mild irritant. The erythema marked with superficial inflammation usually disappear in a few hours but may last for several days, when the upper layer of the skin peels off but leaves no scars.

Second degree- This comprises acute inflammation and formation of blister produced by the prolonged application of flames, liquid at a boiling point or solid much above the boiling point of water. Blisters can be produced by the application of strong irritant of vesicants, such as cantharides. Blisters may also be produced on the part of the body which is allowed to soak in a decomposing fluid, such as urine or faeces & subject to warmth, as seen in old bed-ridden patients.

DERMO EPIDERMAL

Third degree- This refers to the destruction of the cuticles & part of the true skin. Exposure of nerve endings gives rise to much pain. This leaves a scar, but no contraction, as the scar contains all the elements of the true skin.

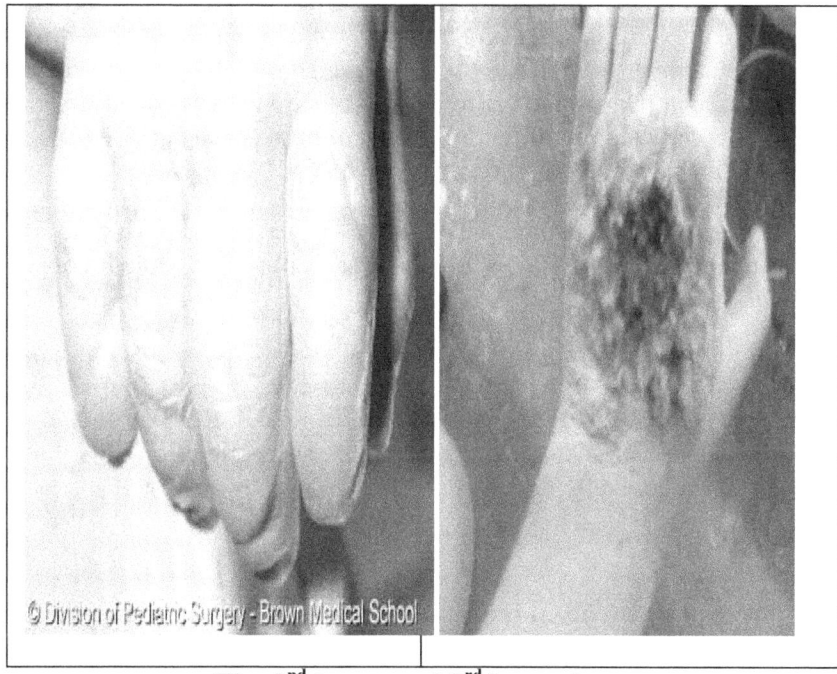

Fig: 2nddegree and 3rddegree burn

Fourth degree- The whole skin is destroyed. There is coagulation necrosis of epidermis & dermis. The lesions have a dry white leathery appearance. The necrosed tissue separates within about a week leaving an ulcer with scar formation. The burns are not very painful as the nerve endings are completely destroyed.

DEEP

Fifth degree- This includes the penetration of the deep fascia & implication of the muscles & results in great scarring and deformity.

Sixth degree- This involves charring of the whole limb including the bones & ends in inflammation of the subjacent tissues and organs.

EFFECTS OF BURNS

❖ **The intensity of the heat applied-** The effects are much more severe of the heat applied is very great.

❖ **The duration of exposure-** The symptoms are also more severe, if the application of heat is continued for a long time.

❖ **The extent of total body surface area-** The surface area burnt is more important than the degree of burn in assessing prognosis of a given case. As for example a first degree burn over a wide area is more dangerous than a third degree burn over a limited area. Destruction of one third of skin area is usually fatal though instant are known when victim with 80 percent burns have survived with skilled treatment when appropriate facilities are available.

❖ **The site-** Burns on the trunk, head, neck & genitals are said to be more dangerous than on other parts of the body, on account of possible involvement of vital structures.

❖ **Age-** Infants, young children & the elderly are particularly vulnerable to initial shock & subsequent complication.

❖ **The sex-** Sensitive & nervous women are more susceptible to burns than strong women & women generally do not bear burns so well as men.

CAUSES OF DEATH

❖ **Shock-** Severe pain & marked protein rich fluid loss from extensive burns which results in increased capillary permeability caused shock and produce a feeble pulse, pale & cold skin, hypotension and collapse, resulting in death instantaneously or within 24 to 48 hours. Shock may also occur from fright before the individual is affected by burns if his heart is weak or diseased.

❖ **Suffocation-** Persons removed from houses destroyed by fire are often found from suffocation due to the inhalation of smoke, carbon dioxide and carbon monoxide- the products of combustion. In such case burns found on the body are usually of post- mortem.

❖ **Accidents or injuries-** Death may result from an accident occurring in an attempt to escape from a burning house or from injuries inflicted by walls and timbers falling on the body.

- **Inflammation-** Inflammation of serous membrane and internal organs, such as meningitis, peritonitis, edema glottidis, pleurisy, bronchitis, broncho pneumonia, pneumonia, enteritis & perforating ulcer of the duodenum.

- **Exhaustion-** Exhaustion from suppurative discharges lasting for weeks or months.

FATAL PERIOD

Death may occur within 24 to 48 hours, but usually the first week is the most fatal.

In suppurative cases death may occur after five or six weeks or even longer.

POST MARTEM APPEARANCES

External-

- The articles of clothing, if any on the body, should be removed very carefully and examined for the presence of characteristic smell of kerosene, petrol or some other combustible substances. They should be returned to the police in a sealed packed especially in murder cases.

- The external appearances of burns vary according to the nature of the substances used to produce them. Thus, the skin is whitened when a burn has been caused by radiant heat.

- Burns produced by flamed may or may not produced blisters but singeing of the hair, eye brows & blackening of the skin are always present.

- Burns caused by explosions in coal mines or of gunpowder are usually very extensive and are accompanied by blackening & tattooing due to the driving of particles of unexploded powder into the skin.

- Burns caused by kerosene oil are usually very severe and are known from its characteristic odour & the sooty blackening of the parts.

- When a body has been exposed to great heat, it gets cooked and becomes so rigid with the limbs fixed, arms fixed & fingers hooked like claws that it assumes an altitude of defense called the "pugilistic" or "fencing" posture. It is due to heat stiffening.

Internal-

- The skull bones are found fractured or burst open, if intense heat been applied, characteristic curved fractures in skull and long bones are reported. The brain and its meninges are generally congested.

- There is extravasation of the blood, usually brick red or a reddish brown deposit upon the upper surface of the duramater.
- The brain is sometimes shrunken, though its form is retained. Sometimes if the head is exposed to severe heat after death not only the charred skull vault may be fractured causing false suspicion of violence but there is a thin layer of extradural blood underneath, which looks like a cooked spongy mass. This has been called a heat haemotoma.
- If death has occurred from suffocation, the nasopharynx, trachea and bronchial tubes may contain sooty carbon particles, and their mucous membrane may be congested and covered with frothy mucus, the absence of soot indicates that the deceased was not alive at the time of fire.
- Some of the sooty mucous may trickle into the stomach.
- The spleen is enlarged & softened. The liver may show cloudy swelling and necrosis of the cells, seen mostly in cases treated with tannic acid, if death has been delayed.

Medicolegal Aspect of Burns

Antemortem & Postmortem

A person may be murdered & heat may be applied to the dead body to conceal the crime. It is therefore necessary to know the differentiating features of antemortem from postmortem. The differentiation depends on presence of a vital reaction as seen by naked eye or by histological examination. In both cases the medical officer should be prepared to tell the difference between antemortem and postmortem burns.

Antemortem

- An antemortem burn shows redness of the parts. In the case of a burn caused during life a line of redness involving the whole true skin is formed round about the injured part.
- It is a permanent line, persisting even after death, but redness or erythema, which is found beyond this line of redness due to distension of the capillaries, is transient, disappear under pressure during life and fades after death.
- The of redness, being a vital function, separates living from dead tissue, and is always present in burns caused during life, though it take some time to appear.
- Hence it is possible that it may be absent in the case of a person of a very weak constitution who dies immediately from shock due to burns.

- ❖ If vesicles are present caused by a burn during life contains a serous fluid consisting of albuminous fluid, chlorides & often a few polymorphonuclear white blood cells and has a red, inflamed base with raised papillae.
- ❖ The skin surrounding it is of a bright red or coppery colour. This is known as true as compared with false vesication which is produced after death.
- ❖ False vesication contains air only but may contain a very small quantity of serum comprising a trace of albumen, but not chlorides as in a person suffering from general anascara.
- ❖ When a vesicle contains pus, it means that the person has lived for at least 36 hours after the injury.

Postmortem

- ❖ A postmortem blister is limited in size, contains air, or if it contains fluid, this is practically non albuminous & does not contain chlorides and blood corpuscles, there is no line of hyperaemia round the blister and its base is not injected.
- ❖ Blister may also be seen in putrefaction but these differ from antemortem blister by the absence of a vital reaction, elevation of entire epidermis from corium to form the covering of the blister and the presence in the blister mainly of putrefactive gases and of a little reddish coloured fluid.
- ❖ Such blisters do not contain any albuminous fluid or chlorides.
- ❖ In case of doubt, it is best to excise the vesicle and its related tissue and examine histologically for evidence of a tissue reaction.

The differentiating features of **ANTEMORTEM** from **POSTMORTEM BURNS** are tabulated:

		ANTEMORTEM BURNS	POSTMORTEM BURNS
1.	**Line of redness**	Present	Absent
2.	**Vesicles**	Contain albuminous fluid & chlorides	Contain air

3.	**Infection**	Pus & sloughing	Nil
4.	**Healing**	Granulation	Nil
5.	**Soot in upper Respiratory tract**	Present	Absent
6.	**Carbohaemoglobin In blood**	Present	Absent
7.	**Enzymes**	Increase in enzymes	No such increase

Burning as a Cause of Death

The presence of antemortem blisters, finding of particles of soot in air passages, oesophagus, and stomach, and cherry red colour of blood due to presence of carbon monoxide are certain signs of death from burning as a result of a conflagration. Their absence suggests some other cause.

SUICIDE, HOMICIDE, OR ACCIDENT

❖ Once the medical officer determines that the cause of death is thermal burns with or without inhalation of toxic products of combustion, the manner of death inevitably will be a matter of careful evaluation of the scene and circumstances of death.

❖ If the individual stood in full view in a public place, poured petrol on his clothing, and then lit a match, the manner of death would clearly be suicide.

❖ However, if identical remains are recovered from a building which has been deliberately set on fire by another than the manner of death would be homicide.

❖ The distribution of burns in most cases is extremely important in relation to the manner of death.

❖ Consider for a moment the case of a burnt child. The police may feel that the child has been abused while the parents claimed that the child crawled i8nto the hot water.

194

❖ If the child has been abused by holding its wrists and ankles and then dipped in hot water, sparing of hands and feet with severe burning of the buttocks will results.

SUICIDAL BURNING

❖ It is relatively common among the Indian women, mostly on account of domestic worries, cruelty by the husband and in-laws, or because of the problem of dowry or some disease.
❖ In suicide, the circumstances are usually evident and perhaps the most frequent method of doing this is to soak the clothes in kerosene and then to set them on fire.
❖ It is difficult to extinguish such flames. Sometimes, suicidal burning is resorted to as a mode of public protest.

HOMICIDAL BURNING

❖ It is rare but cases are recorded where fire, kerosene, petrol, hot metals, and corrosive substances have been used with criminal intent.
❖ Homicidal cases are fairly common in India mainly due to suspected infidelity of the woman or inadequate dowry.
❖ Among adult females, burns are produced usually on the pudenda as a punishment for adultery.
❖ The body may then be burnt to conceal the crime. The battering of children in the west may not always be by mechanical violence and a variety of thermal injuries have been reported.
❖ Deliberate focal lesions from cigarettes and burning of buttocks and other areas on hot plates and radiator bars are examples of this form of child abuse.
❖ If such injuries have occurred at different times suggesting repetitive child abuse, the diagnosis is more certain.

SCALDS

❖ A scald is an injury resulting from application of liquid at or near boiling point, or in its gaseous form, such as steam.

❖ In such cases, only the superficial layers of the skin are affected. The severity of injury depends primarily on the temperature and duration of contact. Burns result in 20 second at 131 degree F, 3 second at 140 degree F, 2 degree F & 1 second at 158 degree F.Almost all scald burns caused by inadvertent turning of hot water tap could be avoided if the setting of hot water heater does not exceed 120 degree F.

- ❖ Scalds are usually not so severe as burns, they mostly produce hyperaemia and vesiculation, as the liquids producing them run off the surface of the body, and rapidly cool on accounts of their evaporation, but they resemble burns very much in severity, when produced by oils or other sticky substances, when boil at a much higher temperature.
- ❖ Scalds produced by molten metals cause great destruction of the affected tissues, as they adhere to the part struck.
- ❖ The liquid responsible for scalding may be seen on clothes and body. Sometimes, its smell may be obvious. The skin is saddened and bleached in appearances.
- ❖ Vesication (Blistering) is an important feature. Vesicles are abundant along the course of the running liquid. The clothes, singeing of the hairs deposition of carbonaceous material and charring of tissues (Common in burns) are not seen.
- ❖ Since the hot fluid or steam is cooled during its passage through the clothing the distribution of the scalds is normally on unclothed parts of the body.
- ❖ Scars of scalds are much thinner than those of buns and cause much less contraction and disfigurement.

Scalds are classified in 3 degrees:

Reddening of skin (Erythema)

- ❖ Redness appears at once and blistering takes place within a few minutes.
- ❖ The blisters are surrounded by a thin bright red area of inflammation.
- ❖ There is reddening & swelling of the papilla in the floor of the blister.
- ❖ If the blistered skin is removed it will leave a pink raw surface.
- ❖ If super heated steam is inhaled, the mucosa of larynx & trachea may be necrosed & detached in shreds.
- ❖ Laryngeal oedema may be responsible for death.

Blister formation

(Vesication due to increased capillary permeability).

- ❖ An antemortem burn shows redness of the parts. If Vesication is present, blisters are surrounded by a thin bright red area of inflammation they contain highly albuminous fluid, chlorides and blood corpuscles.
- ❖ A postmortem blister is limited in size, contains air, or if it contains and blood corpuscles there is no line of hyperaemia round the blister and its bases not injected. Blisters may also be seen in putrefaction but these differ from antemortem blister by the absence of vital reaction, elevation of entire epidermis

Necrosis of the dermis (Deeper layer of skin)

Scalds are usually accidental due to splashing of fluid from cooking utensils or pouring hot water during bath.

❖ Children may upset the vessels containing boiling liquids or suck the spouts of kettles containing hot milk or tea resulting in severe scalds of mouth & throat.
❖ Boiling water may be thrown with intent to injure or annoy.
❖ Deliberate scalding by hot fluid is common in child abuse.

Distinguishing features of burns from dry heat, moist heat & chemicals:

		DRY HEAT	MOIST HEAT	CHEMICAL
1.	Cause	Flame, heated solid substance or radiant heat	Steam or any liquid at or near boiling point	Corrosive acids and alkalis
2.	Site	At and above the site of flame	At and above the site of contact	At and below the site of contact
3.	Clothing	Burnt and may be adherent to the body	Usually wet but not burnt	Characteristic stains
4.	Skin	Dry shriveled, charred	Sodden and bleached	Stained, corroded
5.	Vesicles	At circumference of burnt area	Most marked over burnt area	Rarely found
6.	Red line	Present	Present	Absent
7.	Singeing	Present	Absent	Absent
8.	Charring	Present	Absent	In case of mineral acids
9.	Trickle marks	Absent	Present	Present

10.	Discolouration	Skin roasted and charred	Skin bleached	From action of chemical on skin
11.	Ulceration	Absent	Absent	Present
12.	Scar	Thick and causes disfigure	Thin and causes less disfigurement	Keloid scar and much disfigurement

References:

1. Basu S.C. , Hand Book Of Forensic Medicine and Toxicology, *third edition (2007),* Current Distributors, Lenin Saranee, Calcutta.(page 45 to 50).
2. Modi. Jaising. P, Textbook of Medical Jurisprudence And Toxicology, Twenty *First Edition (1997),* N.M. Tripathi Private Limited, Bombay.

Chapter 17

IMPOTENCE AND STERILITY

IMPOTENCE AND STERILITY

IMPOTENCE: It is defined as physical incapacity or inability to perform sexual intercourse.

FRIGIDITY: It is psychological fault with the female having an abnormal antipathy to sexual intercourse.[1]

FERTILITY: It is opposite of sterility. It means the ability to procreate or conceive children.[2]

STERILITY: It means inability on the part of male to procreate and on the part of the female to conceive children.[3]

STERILIZATION: It is a procedure of making a person infertile without interfering with his or her potency.

MALE IMPOTENCY:

SYNONYM: Erectile Dysfunction

DEFINITION: Male impotency can be defined as inability of a man to achieve and maintain an erection sufficient for mutually satisfactory intercourse with partner.[1]

TYPES OF IMPOTENCY:[1]

- Temporary causes
- Permanent or organic causes

CAUSES OF IMPOTENCY:[1]

➢ In extreme of age, impotency is seen.
➢ Usually, any disease can cause impotency by altering the nervous, vascular and hormonal systems. Many diseases causes change in the smooth muscles of penis causing impotence.

EXAMINATION OF CASE OF IMPOTENCY:[1]

- Informed consent: to avoid embarrassment.
- Details of history of illness: especially with reference to nervous and mental conditions and his sexual history.[8]
- Details of history of medication: any drug that can lead to impotency, like Diazepam which is an anti-depressant.
- Details of history of surgery
- General physical examination: leading to systemic examination.
- Systemic examination: special attention should be directed to nervous and an assessment of mental conditions.[8]
- Local examination for :
  - i. Injuries
  - ii. Malformation related to genital tract
  - iii. Conditions of genital organs (testes, epididymis ,cord ,penis)
  - iv. Length of penis (mons to tip of glans)
     Usually the axis of erect penis horizontally ranges $16°$ to $36°$

MEDICOLEGAL IMPORTANCE:[1,2]

- ❖ Nullity of marriage [1,2]
- ❖ Divorce[1,2]
- ❖ An alleged accused of disputes paternity and rape may claim to be impotent.[1,2]
- ❖ Compensation may be asked for causing impotence.[1]

POTENCY TESTS:

1. **Semen analysis** to evaluate certain characteristics of a male's semen to know male fertility.[1]
2. **Penile Doppler Ultrasound** to know how much and how well blood flows into and out of the penis. This test can tell which direction blood is flowing. For an erection , blood must flow into the penis , but not flow out.[1]
   Venous Leak Syndrome , is a condition in which viens do not "shut off" at the right time, so too much blood flows out of the penis, and the erection is not firm.
   Also, erectile dysfunction can be caused by nerve damage , like in **diabetes**.[1]

3. **Visual erection examination** of penis is carried out in both states , aroused and flaccid , to check for any sort of dysfunction or damage. Morning erection of accused is also important to be tested.[1]

STERILITY

- It is an inability of a male or female to procreate.[1]

- It is a state of being unable to produce offsprings.[1]

- In female , it is inability to conceive.[1]

- In males ,it is an inability to impregnate.[1]

TYPES OF STERILITY OR INFERTILITY:

- Primary
- Secondary

Primary Infertility:

When a couple have never had children, or have been unable to achieve pregnancy, even after living together for more than 1 year, and despite having unprotected sexual intercourse.[1]

Secondary Infertility:

When a couple have had children or achieved pregnancy previously, but are unable to conceive this time, despite having 1 year of unprotected sexual intercourse.[1]

EXAMINATION OF CASE OF STERILITY:[3]

- In a male, the semen is examined.

It is desirable for him to abstain from coitus for a week.

The sample is obtained by masturbation or prostatic massage and examined within 2 hours for spermatozoa.

- In females, attention is directed to development of uterus, and patency of fallopian tubes.

Any defect of vagina is likely to be obvious.

An opinion can be given on the basis of available findings.[3]

CAUSES OF STERILITY:

- o Causes of male sterility
- o Causes of female sterility

Causes of male impotency and sterility:[1,2,3,4,6]

1. **Age:** as age advances, sexual fitness and power gradually diminishes, also, sperm motility is reduced.
2. **Malformations:**
   - Partial or complete absence or loss of penis.
   - Severe forms of hypospadius & epispadius.
   - Absence or loss of both the testicles.
   - Cryptorchids ,i.e., person with undescended testis may occasionally be sterile but, not impotent.
   - Severe form of urethral fistula.
3. **Local injuries or diseases:**
   - Mumps
   - Syphilis
   - Cancer
   - Tuberculosis
   - Elephantiasis of scrotum or penis.
   - Testicular atrophy
4. **General diseases :**
   - Diabetes mellitus, albuminuria , T.B may produce temporary impotence.
   - Endocrine disorders and chromosomal abnormalities.
   - Certain diseases of brain & spinal cord (like paraplegia)
   - Injury to head or spinal cord causing damage to lumbar centre may cause impotency.
5. **Injuries & addictions:**

Injury by occupational exposure to lead, exposure to x-rays.

Chronic alcoholism and abuse of narcotics such as opium may lead to sterility.

6. **Psychic causes :**
    o   Fear
    o   Too much passion for a particular woman and aversion for others may produce temporary impotency.

Impotence quoad hanc: is a condition in a male who may be impotent with a particular woman (may be his wife) but not with other woman (may be a prostitute).[2]

7. **Operations:** Surgeries involving penis , scrotum, prostrate or pelvis may cause nerve damage.[3]

Causes for female sterility:

1. **Age** : as age advances fertility in women decreases, especially over 35years of age.[1]
2. Blockage of fallopian tubes.[1]
3. **Ovulation disorders** : disorders in hypothalamus-pituitary-ovarian system,etc.[1,2]
4. **Uterine factors :** [1]
    ▪   Congenital malfunctions
    ▪   Fibroids
    ▪   Adhesion of uterus due to infection.
5. **Cervical factors** : in some cases cervical is so narrow that it prevents the passage of sperm into the uterus.[1]
6. **Vaginal factors** : rarely, conditions like vaginal septum that inhibits sperm transportation and even the congenital absence of vagina, can be a cause of sterility.[1]
7. **Extreme spasm of vaginal muscles** : like in vaginismus , during intercourse can prevent penetration of penis , and so results in infertility.[1,2]
8. **Surgery** : hysterectomy, ligature of both fallopian tubes.[4]
    MEDICO LEGAL IMPORTANCE:[1]
    ➢   Disputed paternity

> ➢ Compensation cases
> ➢ Sterility can be taken as a plea for adopting a child.

STERILIZATION

This is a procedure which renders a person (male or female) sterile without any interference with potency .[6]

TYPES OF STERILIZATION:[1]

> ➢ Voluntary sterilization
> ➢ Compulsory sterilization

Voluntary sterilization:

Usually undertaken by married couples for the purpose of birth control.

Compulsory sterilization:

This procedure is carried out in some countries, but not in India.[1]

Compulsory sterilization, also known as **forced sterilization**, programs are government policies in violation of human rights conventions which attempt to force people to undergo surgical or other sterilization. The reasons governments implement sterilization programs vary in purpose and intent.

METHODS OF STERILIZATION:[1]

> ★ Temporary
> ★ Permanent

MEDICO LEGAL IMPORTANCE:[1]

> • Legitimacy of child
> • Divorce
> • Disputed paternity

ARTIFICIAL INSEMINATION

> ❖ It is artificial introduction of semen into vagina, cervix or uterus to bring about pregnancy.[6]
> ❖ The usual practice is to deposit 1ml of semen just above the internal or by means of a sterile syringe, at or about the time of ovulation, that is , 14th day after menstruation.[3]

❖ The semen should be collected by masturbation , preferably after a week's abstinence, and used within about 2 hours.[3]

ARTIFICIAL INSEMINATION[9]

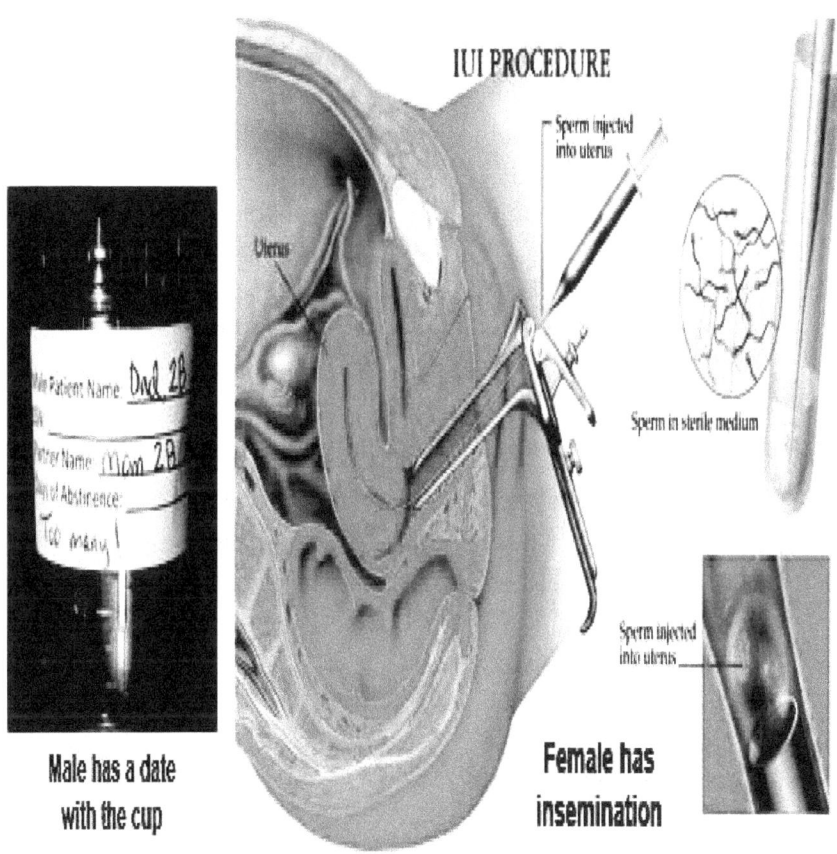

IUI PROCEDURE

Male has a date with the cup

Female has insemination

TYPES OF ARTIFICIAL INSEMINATION:

Artificial Insemination Homologous (AIH) :
It is when the semen of husband of the woman is used.[1,6]

Artificial Insemination Heterologous / Donor (AID) :
When semen of some other person and not the husband of woman is used.[1,6]

INDICATIONS OF ARTIFICIAL INSEMINATION:[1,4]
◈ Incurable defects in husband's semen.[4]

205

- ◈ Husband is sterile.[1]
- ◈ Rhesus incompatibility.[1]
- ◈ Husband is impotent and impotency can't be treated.[4]
- ◈ Hostile vaginal secretions of wife.[1]

LEGAL PRECAUTIONS OF AID:[1,7]

- ❖ Husband and wife must agree , and their consent should be taken in written.[1]
- ❖ Consent from donor's wife.[1,7]
- ❖ Race and characteristics of donor should resemble to that of husband.[1]
- ❖ Donor should be healthy , potent and below the age of 40years.[7]
- ❖ There should be no Rh incompatibility between donor & recipient.[1,7]
- ❖ Blood group of donor should be same as that of husband.[1]
- ❖ Identity of donor as well as recipient should not be disclosed to each other.[7]
- ❖ Donor should not suffer from any hereditary or physical or mental diseases or STD's.[7]
- ❖ Birth certificate should reflect that the husband is the father of child , even though there is no biological connection between husband and child.[1]

MEDICO LEGAL IMPORTANCE:[1]

- • Adultery: donor and recipient are not held guilty of adultery.
- • Legitimacy: As the husband is not the father of the child, so the child will be illegitimate and adoption should be needed.
- • Danger of litigation
- • Nullity of marriage and divorce
- • Incest: risk of incest is more
- • Posthumous child

References:

1. Mahanta Putul (2014) : Modern Textbook of Forensic Medicine & Toxicology , Jaypee Brothers Medical publishers (P) Ltd ,first edition, p.372-377

2. Gupta A.K (2006) : Essentials of Forensic Medicine and Toxicology , Current Distributers , third edition , Kolkata, p. 151-152

3. Parikh C.K (2000) : Parikh's Textbook of Medical Jurisprudence , Forensic Medicine & Toxicology , CBS Publishers & Distributers , sixth edition , p. 5.1-5.7

4. Modi N.J (1983) : Medical Jurisprudence & Toxicology , N.M Tripathi Private Ltd , p. 303-309

5. Usmani Hammad (1976) : Tib-ul-qanoon , Israar Kareemi Press, Allahabad , p.237-238

6. Basu S.C (2007) : Handbook of Forensic Medicine and Toxicology , Current Distributers, fourth edition , Kolkata, p. 117-120

7. Karmakar R.N (2010) : Forensic Medicines and Toxicology , Academic publishers, Kolkata, p. 428-429

8. Vij Krishna (2008) : Textbook of Forensic Medicine & Toxicology: Principles & Practice , Elsevier India , p.52

9. http://www.advancedfertility.com/images/IUI-picture.jpg

Chapter 18

PREGNANCY

PREGNANCY

Pregnancy

Pregnancy is a condition which occurs in the female when she carries a fertilized ovum within the uterus. It is likely to occur during the period between puberty and menopause.

The signs of pregnancy in the living can be divided into

1. Presumptive signs
2. Probable signs
3. Positive or conclusive signs

SIGNS OF PREGNANCY

1. Presumptive Signs

- ❖ Amenorrhea
- ❖ Morning sickness
- ❖ Sympathetic changes
- ❖ Breast changes
- ❖ Chadwick's sign
- ❖ Urinary disturbances
- ❖ Quickening
- ❖ Pigmentation of skin

2. Probable Signs

- ❖ Enlarged abdomen
- ❖ Hegar's sign
- ❖ Goodell's sign
- ❖ Palmer's sign
- ❖ Osiander's sign
- ❖ Piskacek's sign

- ❖ Braxton-hick's sign
- ❖ Uterine soufflé
- ❖ Ballottement
- ❖ Immunological tests
- ❖ Biology tests

3. Positive Signs

- ❖ Fetal movement and parts
- ❖ Fetal heart sounds
- ❖ Radiographs
- ❖ Ultrasonography
- ❖ Fetal cell in mother's blood

Presumptive signs

__Suppression of menstruation/ amenorrhea:__

Menstruation normally ceases after impregnation and does not recur until some months after child birth. However, instances are known of women who have never menstruated becoming pregnant, and menstruation continuing during early months of pregnancy. Again, cessation of menses may result from ill- health, intense desire for pregnancy, or fear of pregnancy after illicit intercourse.

__Morning sickness:__

This often only amounts to nausea and occasionally vomiting which takes places on getting up in the morning. It is usually marked in a primigravida. Though a frequent phenomenon in the early stage of pregnancy yet it is of no great significance, as it is often caused by other conditions, as foe example migraine, ascariasis, gastritis, etc.

__Sympathetic disturbances:__

Salivation, perverted appetite, and irritability of temper mat occur and are caused reflexly by pregnancy. Even minor exertion causes fatigue.

__Change in breasts:__

Change are quite characteristic in primigravidas, but are lesser value in multiparas. Tenseness and tingling in the breasts is evidently by 6-8th week. The nipples become deeply pigmented and more erectile and the areola becomes dark-brown.

- Around the nipple, the sebaceous glands become enlarged (montgomery's tubercles) by the end of 3rd month.
- Colostrum (thin, yellowish fluid) is secreted as early as 12th week which becomes thick and yellow by 16th week.
- Secondary areola, especially in primigravida usually appears by 20th week.
- After 6th month, silvery lines or striae are seen, especially in primiparae due to the stretching of the skin.

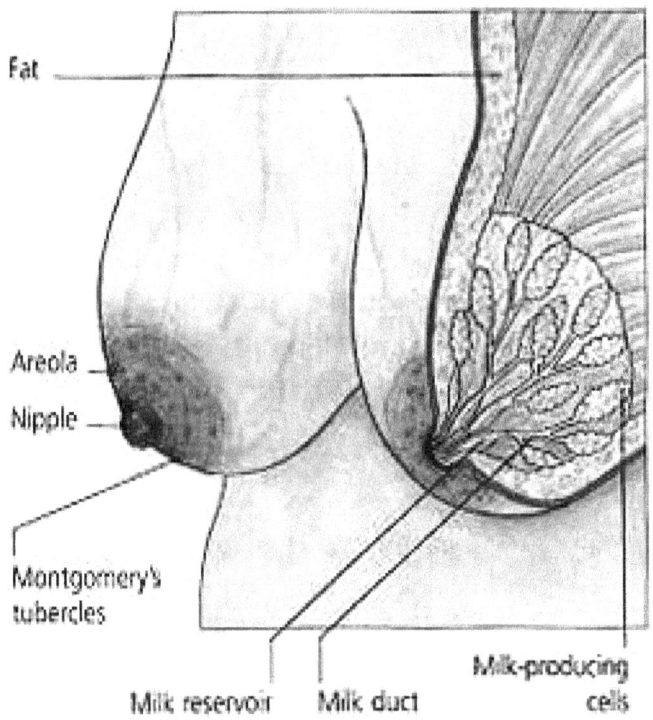

**Jackquemier's or Chadwick's sign:**

These are due to increased vascularity and venous stasis due to pressure of the gravid uterus after the fourth month.these changes form the basis of Jackquemier's sign.(1)The mucous membrane of the vagina changes from pink to violet, deepening to blue as result of venous obstruction at about 8th week of pregnancy.

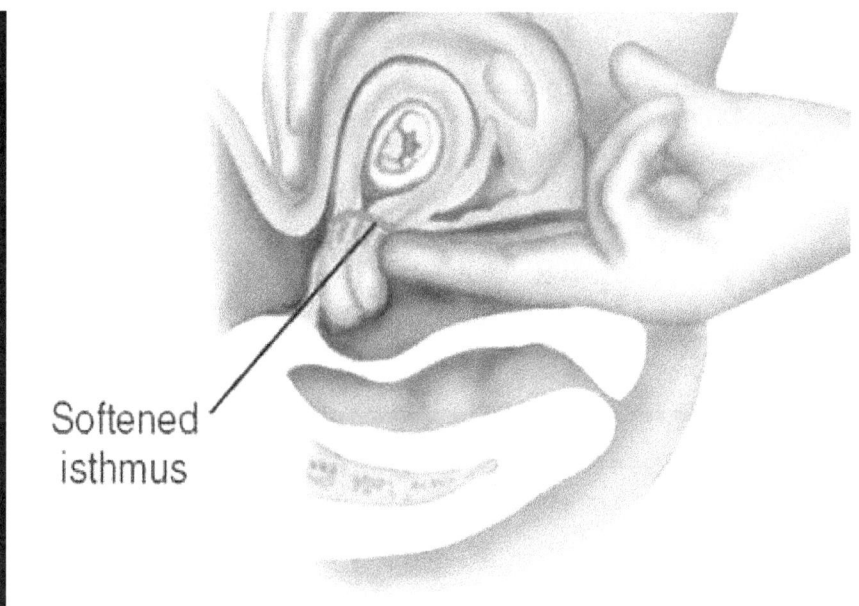

Softened isthmus

Urinary disturbances:

During 8-12th week of pregnancy, the enlarging uterus exerts pressure on the bladder and produces frequent micturition. This gradually disappears after 2th week as the uterus straightens up into the abdomen and reappears a few weeks before term when the head descends into the pelvis.

Quickening:

This is the mother's subjective sensation of the movements of the foetus and occurs at about four to four and half months.

PROBABLE SIGNS OF PREGNANCY:

1. *Enlargement of the abdomen (fundal height):*

During pregnancy, abdomen gradually enlarges in size after the 12th week .during the last two months, the uterus sinks into the pelvis and tends to fall forward due to its weight.

Uterus feels soft and elastic and becomes ovoid in shape which changes to spherical shape beyond 36th week.

The umbilicus becomes level with the skin by about the 7th month.

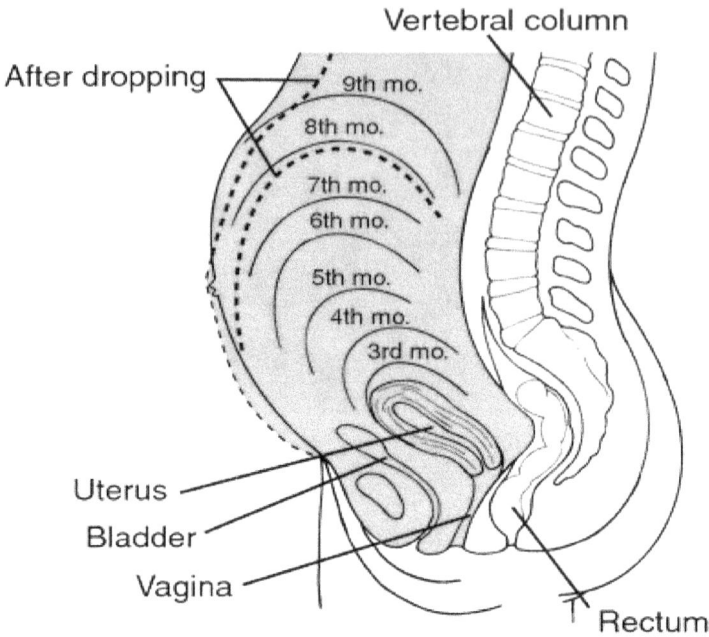

2. *Hegar's sign:*

This is positive between the 6-10th week.

Demonstration: if one hand is placed on the abdomen and two fingers of other hand in the vagina, the firm hand cervix is felt and above it the elastic body of the uterus, while between the two, isthmus is felt as a soft compressible area. This is the most valuable physical sign of early pregnancy.

3. Goodell's sign:

As early as 6th week, the cervix progressively softens from below upward. Pregnant woman's cervix feels like lips and non-pregnant woman's like the tip of the nose. The cervical orifice, during the last months of pregnancy, becomes circular instead of being transverse and admits the point of finger to greater depth.

4. Palmer's sign:

Regular rhythmic contractions of uterus can be elicited by bimanual examination as early as 4-6th week.

5. **Osiander's sign:**

There is an increased pulsation felt through the lateral fornices at about 8th week.

6. **Piskacek's sign:**

Asymmetrical enlargement of uterus occurs, the there is lateral implantation. Here on half of uterus is more firm that the other.

7. **Braxton-hick's contraction:**

Intermittent, spasmodic, painless uterine contractions are observed rarely before the 3rd month, but are easily felt after the 4th month. Each contraction lasts for about a minute and relaxation for about 2-3 min.

8. **Ballottement (loss up like a ball):**

This is posiive during the 4th-5th month of pregnancy as the fetus is small in relation to the amount of amniotic fluid present.

9. *Uterine souffle:*

It is soft blowing murmur, which is synchronous with the mother's pulse .it is heard towards the end of 4th month by auscultation, on either side of the uterus (due to passage of blood through the uterine vessels)just above inguinal ligament.

10. **Biological tests:**
   These are based on the reaction of test animals to human chorionic gonadotropins (hcg) in the pregnant woman's serum or urine.
   The tests are:
   (1) Aschheim-zondek test (classical biological test)
   (2) Rapid rat test
   (3) Freidman test or female rabbit test
   (4) Hogben or female toad test
   (5) Galli-manini test or male frog test (most popular biological test)
11. **Immunological tests:**

hcG can be detected in maternal serum / urine by 8-11days after conception (maximum level is reached in 10-11 weeks). The test is not reliable after 12 weeks .the advantages of the tests are:

a) Convenient and sensitive (accuracy 98%)
b) No animal is required
c) Results are quicker (2min)

Immunological tests have replaced biological tests for routine screening the highest level of hCG and is preferable for testing.

Limitation:: it will give positive test with ectopic pregnancy, hydatidiform mole and choriocarcinoma.

POSITIVE SIGNS

1. **Fetal movement:** fetal movement and fetal parts can be identified distinctly by 20th week on abdominal palpation.

2. **Fetal heart sounds:** definite sign of pregnancy. They are heard beteen 18-20th week with an ordinary stethoscope. The sound are like thethiking of a watch placed under a pillow. The rrate is usually about 160/min at 5th month and 140/min at 9th month, and is not synchronous with the mother's pulse.

3. Uterine souffle and fetal (due to inrush of blood through umbilical arteries) may be confused with fetal heart sound.

4. **Radiographic imaging**: the earliest fetal skeletal shadow of vertebral dots is visible at about 16th week of pregnancy. The shadows to be searched in the pelvis of the mother are :
   • Series of small dots in linear arrangement of the vertebral column
   • Crescentic or annular shadows of the skull
   • Series of fine curved parallel lines of the ribs
   • Linear shadows of the limb

5. **Ultrasonography:** intra- decidual gestational sac is identified as early as 29-35 days of gestation. Gestational sac and yolk sac by 5th menstrual week, fetal pole and embryonic movement by 7th week.

Transvaginalsonography(tvs) can detect cardiac activity by 5th week and transabdonimal sonography by 6th week. Doppler ultrasound can pick up the fetal rate reliable by 10th week.

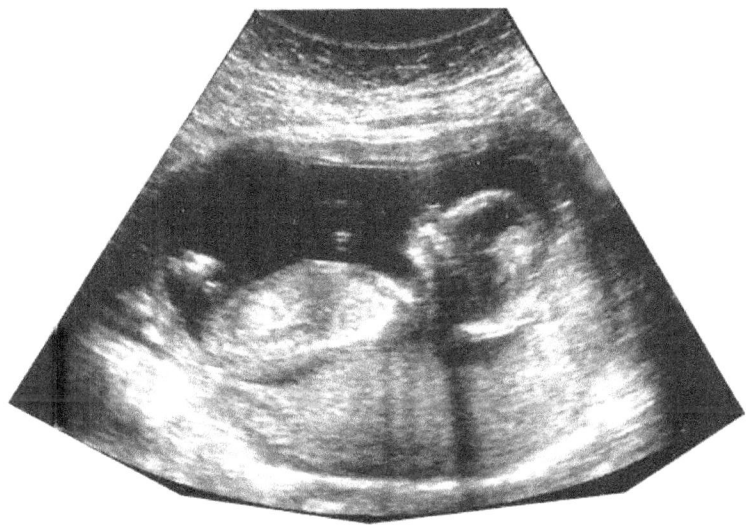

6. **Fetal cells in mother's blood:** it can be detected by 5th week of pregnancy. Even the sex of the fetus can be determined by karyotyping these cells.

Betke-kleihauer test: this is a staining technique in which fetal cell can be distinguished from adult red cell. A blood smear is prepared from mother's blood and exposed to an acid bath. This removes adult haemoglobin , but not fetal haemoglobin from the red blood cells. Subsequent staining makes fetal cells (containing fetal haemoglobin) appear rose- pink in colour, while adult red blood cells are only seen as "ghosts".

Maximum and minimum period of gestation:

1. The usually accepted average is 280 days from the first day of the menstrual period, so that the actual period of gestation is about 270 days or less.
2. The women may over-carry the fetus to [post maturaityupto a period of 320 days oe even upto 350 days.
3. Expulsion of fetus to be viable, it should be of 210 days gestation.
4. A fetus born after 180 days of gestation may survive, if proper care is taken.

   Diagnosis of pregnancy in the dead

External physical change should be noted. In the internal examination, the following should be looked for;

1. Presence of embryo, fetus, placental tissue or membranes—positive proof of pregnancy.
2. Enlarged and thickened uterus
3. Corpus luteum in ovary—corroborative evidence.

Pseudocyesis (spurious/false/phantom pregnancy)

Definition: it is a psychological disorder where the woman has the false but firm belief that she is pregnant, although no pregnancy exists.

❖ It is generally osrved in infertile females or women nearing menopause, who desire a child intensely.

❖ Most of these women suffer from some form of psychic or hormonal disorder.

❖ Such patients may present with all the subjective symptoms of pregnancy including cessation of menstruation and associated with a considerable increase in the size of the abdomen which may be due to abnormal deposition of fat or due to pathological conditions, like ovarian tumor or ascites.

❖ The women may have secretions from the breasts and intestinal movements which she imagines as fetal movement and may have false labor pains.

❖ Obstetrical examination along with ultrasonography and / or immunological tests for pregnancy will clear the patient of her imagination.

Superfecundation

Definition: fertilization of two ova discharged from ovary at the same period of ovulation by two different acts of coitus committed at short intervals.

❖ The term is also used to refer to instance of two different males fathering fraternal twins, though this is more accurately known as hetropaternal superfecundation. This leads to the possiblility of twins also being half-siblings, classic example being one baby is white and the other black.

❖ Medico-legal aspect: gross variation occur in the complexion and features of the two babies and may give rise to the doubt of adultery and infidelity.

Superfetation

Definition: fertilization of two ova discharged from ovary at different period of ovulation.

- ❖ It is fertilization of second ovum in pregnant woman.
- ❖ In this, one fetus always remains more developed than the other and may be born either at the same time showing different maturation or may born at different period, varying from 1-3 months.
- ❖ Possibility is more with septate or double uterus.

Fetal compressus or papyraceus: In a twin pregnancy, one fetus may grow at the cost of the other, the later may die, flattened by pressure into a mummified parchment- like state known as fetuspapyraeus and may not be orgaizable. It is retained till labor expels it.

Legitimacy and paternity

Definition: it is the legal state of a person born in a lawful marriage.

Legitimate child: person who born during the continuance of legal marriage or within 280days after the dissolution of the marriage by divorce or death of the husband anfd the mother remaining unmarried.

Illegitimate child or bastard: child born out of lawful wedlock or not within a competent time after dissolution of marriage or if it can be proved that the alleged father is:

- ❖ Under the age of puberty
- ❖ Physically incapable to beget children, because of illness, impotence or sterility
- ❖ Not having access sexually to his wife during the time that the child was begotten
- ❖ Having incompatibility of blood groups.

Chapter 19

MEDICAL TERMINATION OF PREGNANCY

MEDICAL TERMINATION OF PREGNANCY (MTP)

Medical Termination of Pregnancy (MTP):

MTP is Medical Termination of Pregnancy. It also called induced abortion. It is the medical way of getting rid of unwanted pregnancy. MTP should always be performed at a place recognized by government authorities.

Abortion is a procedure that enables a woman to opt out of an unwanted pregnancy. Medical procedure for ending a pregnancy at any time before the foetus has attained the stage of viability is called Medical Termination of Pregnancy (MTP) or abortion. It is not a family planning method but it is a reliable method of terminating unplanned and unwanted pregnancy.

An abortion can be induced or spontaneous. A spontaneous abortion occurs when a pregnancy terminates without any medical or surgical intervention, as in the case of a miscarriage. Induced abortions involve surgical or medical procedures for termination of the pregnancy.

Information on who can seek an abortion in India and the procedure involved:

Abortion has been legal in India since 1971, when the Medical Termination of Pregnancy Act was passed. The law is quite liberal, as it aims to reduce illegal abortion and maternal mortality.

Discontinuation of pregnancy has been practiced from time immemorial. The procedure was known to practitioners of Gynecological Medicine but because of society's attitude it has resulted in unnecessary complications. Our Government recognized this silent need in society and passed a legislation called 'The Medical Termination of Pregnancy Act in 1971' which came into force from 1st April, 1972. This act makes the termination of pregnancies legal for doctors and for clients. India is among the first few countries to legalize termination of unwanted pregnancy.

An abortion can be performed in India until the 20th week of pregnancy. The opinion of a second doctor is required if the pregnancy is past its 12th week.

The Medical Termination of Pregnancy Act was amended in 2002 and 2003 to allow doctors to provide **mifepristone** and **misoprostol** (also known as the "**morning-after pill**") on prescription up until the seventh week of pregnancy.

Indications for Medical Termination of Pregnancy

❖ A woman has a serious disease and the pregnancy could endanger her life.

- ❖ A woman's physical or mental health is endangered by the pregnancy.
- ❖ The foetus has a substantial risk of physical or mental handicap
- ❖ A woman contracts rubella (German measles) during the first three months of pregnancy
- ❖ Any of a woman's previous children had congenital abnormalities
- ❖ The foetus is suffering from RH disease
- ❖ The foetus has been exposed to irradiation
- ❖ The pregnancy is the result of rape
- ❖ A woman's socio-economic status may hamper a healthy pregnancy
- ❖ A contraceptive device failed

Permission
- ❖ If a woman is married, her own written consent is sufficient. Her husband's consent is not required
- ❖ If a woman is unmarried and over 18, she can provide her own written consent
- ❖ If a woman is unmarried and under 18, she must provide written consent from her guardian
- ❖ If a woman is mentally unstable, she must provide written consent from her guardian

Medical Termination of Pregnancy is legally permitted up to 20 weeks of gestation. Pregnancy termination performed in first trimester is safer than in second trimester since it has fewer complications. It is illegal to perform MTP after determining sex of the child as Government of India has banned sex determination.

Under the MTP Act, the following are strictly specified:
- ❖ Maternal/ Fetal conditions under which MTP can be done
- ❖ Place where it can be done
- ❖ Persons who can do it

Complications of MedicallyTerminated Pregnancy
Medical Termination of Pregnancy (MTP) is a procedure that is carried out under anesthesia & increases the risk for the procedure. Patient can have lot of bleeding during & after the procedure. There are high chances of patient having recurrent abortions. Rarely, patient may not conceive again if infection sets in.

Procedure
- ❖ Abortions can be performed in any medical institution that is licensed by the government to perform medically assisted terminations of pregnancy. Such institutions must display a certificate issued by the government.

Abortions must be performed by a doctor with one of the following qualifications:
- ❖ A registered medical practitioner who has performed at least 25 medically assisted terminations of pregnancy.
- ❖ A surgeon who has six months' experience in obstetrics and gynecology.
- ❖ A person who has a diploma or degree in obstetrics and gynecology.

- A doctor who was registered before the 1971 Medical Termination of Pregnancy Act and who has three years' experience in obstetrics and gynecology.
- A doctor who registered after 1971 and has been practising in obstetrics and gynecology for at least a year.
- The best way to find a gynecologist is through personal recommendations or by visiting the gynecology and obstetrics department of a reputed private hospital or clinic.
- Indian society is quite conservative and pre-marital sex is taboo. Unmarried women seeking an abortion may be confronted by medical staff with hostile attitudes.

Time Factor in Abortion

An MTP or abortion undertaken for a 10 or 11 weeks old foetus is safe, 12 weeks, which is equal to two and half calendar months, is not a recommended period because now the foetus is neither too small nor too big. After 16 weeks, the MTP needs to be executed like a mini-labour by administering injections that can cause expulsion of the foetus. At this stage, if the injection does not seem to work, the abdomen may need to be opened up and the MTP executed like a caesarian.

It is important to realize that while what you are undergoing is a minor operation, its effects are important. Avoid quacks and neighbourhood clinics altogether. Make sure that you are undergoing the procedure under the hands of a capable doctor and in a clean and reliable hospital.

Precautions

Most women are able to have abortions at clinics or outpatient facilities if the procedure is performed early in pregnancy. Women who have stable diabetes, controlled epilepsy, mild to moderate high blood pressure, or who are HIV positive can often have abortions about patients if precautions are taken. Women with heart disease, previous endocarditis, asthma, lupus erythematosus, uterine fibroid tumors, blood clotting disorders, poorly controlled epilepsy, or some psychological disorders usually need to be hospitalized in order to receive special monitoring and medications during the procedure.

Does a woman require a written consent of her husband to get an MTP done?

A woman can give her own consent if she is above 18 years of age, she does not require the consent of her husband. However a girl below 18 years needs the consent of her guardian in writing.

Where abortion should be performed?

Since making termination of pregnancy legal in 1971, Government has given license to a few well qualified doctors and institutions to conduct termination of pregnancy. Abortion should always be done by these trained and qualified doctors at MTP registered clinics.

Very early abortions

Between five and seven weeks, a pregnancy can be ended by a procedure called menstrual extraction. This procedure is also sometimescalled menstrual regulatio n, minisuction, or premptive abortion.

The contents of the uterus are suctioned out through a thin (3-4 mm) plastic tube that is inserted through the undilated cervix. Suction isapplied either by a bulb syringe or a small pump.

Another method is called the "morning after" pill, or emergency contraception. Basically, it involves taking high doses of birth controlpills within 24 to 48 hours of having unprotected sex. The high doses of hormones cause the uterine lining to change so that it will notsupport a pregnancy. Thus, if the egg has been fertilized, it is simply expelled from the body.

First trimester abortions

The first trimester methods of abortion include:

❖ Cervical dilatation followed by evacuation of uterus by Curettage /Suction evacuation / vacuum aspiration / Dilatation and evacuation.

❖ Menstrual aspiration (MR)

❖ Medical Methods

CERVICAL DILATION FOLLOWED BY EVACUATION-

It is a kind of surgical abortion done in the early pregnancy that is before 12 weeks by first dilating the cervix, which is done by introducing hollow metal rods of increasing diameters and then evacuating the contents of the uterus mechanically by scraping or by suction or both. The procedure takes about 15 minutes.

MENSTRUAL ASPIRATION

The first trimester of pregnancy includes the first 13 weeks after the last menstrual period. In the United States, about 90% of abortions are performed during this period. It is the safest time in which to have an abortion, and the time in which women have the most choice of how the procedure is performed.

The advantages of a first trimester medical abortion are:

❖ The procedure is non-invasive; no surgical instruments are used.

❖ Anesthesia is not required.

❖ Drugs are administered either orally or by injection.

❖ The procedure resembles a natural miscarriage.

❖ Disadvantages of a medical abortion are:

❖ The effectiveness decreases after the seventh week.

❖ The procedure may require multiple visits to the doctor.

❖ Bleeding after the abortion lasts longer than after a surgical abortion.

❖ The woman may see the contents of her womb as it is expelled.

❖ Two different medications can be used to bring about an abortion.

The main drugs in use today are a group of drugs known as prostaglandin which can be used through various routes namely by mouth (**referred to as the Abortion Pill**), by injection intramuscularly /intravenously or vaginally. These drugs are used by themselves or in combination with other drugs.

Methotrexate (Rheumatrex)
- ❖ Works by stopping fetal cells from dividing which causes the fetus to die.
- ❖ On the first visit to the doctor, the woman receives an injection of methotrexate. On the second visit, about a week later, she is givenmisoprostol (Cytotec), an oxygenated unsaturated cyclic fatty acid responsible for various hormonal reactions such as muscle contraction (prostaglandin) that stimulates contractions of the uterus. Within two weeks, the woman will expel the contents of her uterus, ending the pregnancy. A follow-up visit to the doctor is necessary to assure that the abortion is complete.
- ❖ With this procedure, a woman will feel cramping and may feel nauseated from the misoprostol. This combination of drugs is 90-96%effective in ending pregnancy.

Mifepristone (RU486): Which goes by the brand name Mifeprex, works by blocking the action of progesterone, a hormone needed for pregnancy to continue, then stimulates uterine contractions thus ending the pregnancy. It can be taken as much as 49 days after the firstday of a woman's last period. On the first visit to the doctor, a woman takes a mifepristone pill. Two days later she returns and, if the miscarriage has not occurred, takes two misoprostol pills, which causes the uterus to contract. Five percent of women won't need to take misoprostol. After an observation period, she returns home.

Within four days, 90% of women have expelled the contents of their uterus and completed the abortion. Within 14 days, 9597% of women have completed the abortion. A third follow-up visit to the doctor is necessary to confirm through observation or ultrasound that the procedure is complete. In the event that it is not, a surgical abortion is performed. Studies show that 4.5 to 8 percent of women need surgery or a blood transfusion after taking mifepristone, and the pregnancy persists in about 1 percent of women. In this case, surgical abortion is recommended because the fetus may be damaged. Side effects include nausea, vaginal bleeding and heavy cramping. The bleeding is typically heavier than a normal period and may last up to 16 days.

Mifepristone is not recommended for women with ectopic pregnancy, an IUD, who have been taking long-term steroidal therapy, have bleeding abnormalities or on blood-thinners such as Coumadin.

Surgical abortions
First trimester surgical abortions are performed using vacuum aspiration.The pro cedure is also called dilation and evacuation (D & E),suction dilation, vacuum cu rettage, or suction curettage.

Advantages of a vacuum aspiration abortion are:
- ❖ It is usually done as a one-day outpatient procedure.
- ❖ The procedure takes only 10-15 minutes.
- ❖ Bleeding after the abortion lasts five days or less.

❖ The woman does not see the products of her womb being removed.

Disadvantages include:
❖ The procedure is invasive; surgical instruments are used.
❖ Infection may occur.
❖ During a vacuum aspiration, the woman's cervix is gradually dilated by expanding rods inserted into the cervical opening. Once dilated, a tube attached to a suction pump is inserted through the cervix and the contents of the uterus are suctioned out. The procedure is 97-99% effective. The amount of discomfort a woman feels varies considerably. Local anesthesia is often given to numb the cervix, but it does not mask uterine cramping. After a few hours of rest, the woman may return home.

Second trimester abortions

The methods may include medical methods and surgical methods.

Medical methods involve the use of Prostaglandin related drugs, which may be given orally or intravaginally or injected directly into the uterine cavity.

The surgical methods include:
❖ **Aspirotomy:** Similar to Dilatation and Evacuation
❖ **Hysterotomy:** Opening the uterus and removal of foetus
❖ **Hysterectomy:** Removal of the entire uterus.

Although it is better to have an abortion during the first trimester, some second trimester abortions may be inevitable. The results of genetic testing are often not available until 16 weeks. In addition, women, especially teens, may not have recognized the pregnancy or come to terms with it emotionally soon enough to have a first trimester abortion. Teens make up the largest group having second trimester abortions.

Some second trimester abortions are performed as a D & E. The procedures are similar to those used in the first trimester, but a larger suction tube must be used because more material must be removed. This increases the amount of cervical dilation necessary and increases the risk of the procedure. Many physicians are reluctant to perform a D & E this late in pregnancy, and for some women is it not a medically safe option.

The alternative to a D & E in the second trimester is an abortion induced labor. Induced labor may require an overnight stay in a hospital. The day before the procedure, the woman visits the doctor for tests and to either have rods inserted in her cervix to help dilate it or to receive medication that will soften the cervix and speed up labor.

On the day of the abortion, drugs, usually prostaglandins to induce contractions, and a salt water solution, are injected into the uterus. Contractions begin, and within eight to 72 hours the woman delivers the fetus.

Side effects of this procedure include nausea, vomiting, and diarrhea from the prostaglandins, and pain from uterine cramps. Anesthesia of the sort used in childbirth can be given to mask the pain. Many women are able to go home a few hours after the procedure.

Preparation

❖ The doctor must know accurately the stage of a woman's pregnancy before an abortion is performed. The doctor will ask the woman questions about her menstrual cycle and also do a physical examination to confirm the stage of pregnancy. This may be done at an office visit before the abortion or on the day of the abortion. Some states require a waiting period before an abortion can be performed. Others require parental or court consent for a child under age 18 to receive an abortion.

❖ Despite the fact that almost half of all women in the United States have had at least one abortion by the time they reach age 45, abortion is surrounded by controversy. Women often find themselves in emotional turmoil when deciding if an abortion is a procedure they wish to undergo. Preabortion counseling is important in helping a woman resolve any questions she may have about having the procedure.

Aftercare

Regardless of the method used to perform the abortion, a woman will be observed for a period of time to make sure her blood pressure isstable and that bleeding is controlled. The doctor may prescribe antibiotics to reduce the chance of infection. Women who are Rh negative (lacking genetically determined antigens in their red blood cells that produce immune responses) should be given a human Rhimmune globulin (RhoGAM) after the procedure unless the father of the fetus is also Rh negative. This prevents blood incompatibility complications in future pregnancies.

Bleeding will continue for about five days in a surgical abortion and longer in a medical abortion. To decrease the risk of infection, a woman should avoid intercourse and not use tampons and douches for two weeks after the abortion.

A follow-up visit is a necessary part of the woman's aftercare. Contraception will be offered to women who wish to avoid future pregnancies, because menstrual periods normally resume within a few weeks.

Risks

Women who have had an abortion worry that it may affect their ability to conceive or bear a child in the future. They will be relieved to learn that now it is generally believed that a single abortion performed in the first 12 weeks of pregnancy does not pose a threat to future childbearing potential. However, a recent World Health Organization study has shown that women who underwent two or more abortions had a two-to-three times greater chance of miscarriage, premature delivery, or low birth weight infants.

Serious complications resulting from abortions performed before 13 weeks are rare. Of the 90% of women who have abortions in this time period, 2.5% have minor complications that can be handled without hospitalization. Less than 0.5% have complications that require a hospital stay. The rate of complications increases as the pregnancy progresses.

Complications from abortions can include:

❖ uncontrolled bleeding
❖ infection

- ❖ blood clots accumulating in the uterus
- ❖ a tear in the cervix or uterus
- ❖ missed abortion where the pregnancy continues
- ❖ Incomplete abortion where some material from the pregnancy remains in the uterus.
- ❖ Women who experience any of the following symptoms of post-abortion complications should call the clinic or doctor who performed the abortion immediately

Normal results

Usually the pregnancy is ended without complication and without altering future fertility.

Advantages and Disadvantages of medical abortion

Advantages

- ❖ There is a greater than 85% chance of avoiding a surgical abortion.
- ❖ The pregnancy can be terminated as soon as there is a positive pregnancy test. This is earlier than the usual surgical abortion.
- ❖ Aborting the pregnancy at home provides more privacy in some cases.
- ❖ Medical abortion does not use instruments inside the uterus so if it is successful, there is no chance of causing damage to the uterus.

Disadvantages

- ❖ There is a 10-15% chance the abortion will not be effective or complete and a surgical procedure will be needed.
- ❖ The abortion will take at least 1 week and may (very rarely) take as long as 5 weeks to complete.
- ❖ Vaginal bleeding may be prolonged and heavy.
- ❖ Medication side effects (less than 10%) such as headaches, nausea, vomiting, sore mouth, dizziness or rash may occur.
- ❖ The need for several clinic visits, blood tests and possibly ultrasounds.
- ❖ Uncertainty about whether the abortion was a success.
- ❖ Medical abortion appointments cannot always be accommodated at the Women's Health Center.

MTP ACT

The MTP Act if adhered to completely offers complete protection to the medical practitioner from any of the consequences of the IPC. However legal protection is only available conditional to every requirement of the Act being fulfilled Sheriar, J Obs Gyn India, 51(6):25, 2002

The MTP Act (Act No. 34 of 1971)

- ❖ "An Act to provide for the Termination of certain pregnancies by registered medical practioners & for matters connected therewith & incidental thereto"
- ❖ Legislated by the Parliament on August 10th , 1971
- ❖ And the Act was enforced Nationwide from April 1st , 1972
- ❖ Adopted by Kashmir & Mizoram- 1980

Medical Termination of Pregnancy-1971

The Medical Termination of Pregnancy Act, 1971 under this Act, pregnancy can be terminated under the following conditions.

1. **Therapeutic:** When the continuation of pregnancy endangers the life of women or may cause serious injury to the physical or mental health.
2. **Eugenic:** When there is risk of the child being born with serious physical or mental abnormalities.
3. **Humanitarian:** When pregnancy has been caused by rape.
4. **Failure of contraception:** When pregnancy has resulted from the failure of contraceptive methods in case of a married women, which is likely to cause serious injury to her mental health.
5. **Socio-economic:** When social or economic environment, actual or reasonably expected can injury the mother's health.

MTP Act, Rules, Regulations

❖ MTP Act Is an Act of Parliament providing an Overview of Safe abortions and delegating authority to Central & State government
❖ Rules are framed by the Central Government BUT must be ratified by each house of Parliament
❖ Regulations are framed by the State Government & relate to issues involving Opinions , reporting and maintaining secrecy

Legal framework

1. MTP Act
2. Rules
3. Regulation

MTP Act Specifies:

❖ The Indications for legal Terminations
❖ Who can Terminate
❖ The Place where it can be terminated
❖ Last but most imp. Consent requirement

When pregnancy can be terminated???

❖ continuation of pregnancy is a risk to the life of pregnant woman or it can cause grave injury to her physical and mental health
❖ Substantial risk that the child , if born ,would be seriously handicapped due to physical or mental abnormalities
❖ pregnancy caused by rape
❖ failure of contraceptive in married woman

Who Can Terminate a Pregnancy?

Who can perform MTP?

❖ A Registered Medical practitioner (RMP)who has a recognized Medical qualification as defined in clause (b) of Sec 2 of Indian Medical Counsel Act, 1956
❖ Whose name is registered in a state Medical register
❖ Who has training experience as per MTP rules

Experience of RMP-

❖ Up to 12 weeks Gestation only

- ❖ Before the commencement of act experience minimum `3yrs
- ❖ Who is registered in state medical register ---6months of house surgeon ship in gynecology or experience of working in dept of gynecology –1yr
- ❖ A Practitioner who has assisted RMP in 25 cases of Medical termination of pregnancies, at least 5 of which have been performed independently in a hospital established or maintained by govt or a training institute approved for this purpose by the Govt.

Experience and Training Required by a RMP
upto 20 wks
- ❖ PG Degree or Diploma in OB & Gynae
- ❖ Completed 6 months as House Surgeon in OB & Gynae
- ❖ At least one yr experience in dept of ob & Gynae at any hospital that has all facilities

Where pregnancy can be terminated?
PLACE
- ❖ Hospitals established or maintained by the Govt.
- ❖ A Place approved by the Government or DLC constituted by the Govt.

Consent Form C
- ❖ Only the consent of a women is required
- ❖ If Age <18 yrs or a mentally ill patient consent of guardian is required.

MTP Rules
- ❖ Appointed by Govt. and responsible for approval and suspension of Place
- ❖ Chaired by CMO
- ❖ 3-5 members
- ❖ One member should be Gynecologist , surgeon , Anesthetist
- ❖ other members are from local doctors, NGO, Panchayat Raj
- ❖ at least one should be woman

Amendments to MTP rules 2003
- ❖ Detailed the composition and tenure of the DLC
- ❖ Abortion sites approved for

A- Up to 12 weeks

B- 12-20 weeks, facilities and equipments required for two types were detailed.
- ❖ Allowed medical abortion using RU486 and misoprostol by RMP even from site not approved provided the RMP has referral linkage access to an approved place.
- ❖ A non obs gynecologist provider who is trained and certified can provide first trimester abortion.

ABORTION
Definition: Expulsion or extraction from its mother of an embryo or fetus weighing 500gm or less when it is not capable of independent (WHO).

Type of abortion
Spontaneous
- ❖ Threatened

227

❖ Inevitable
❖ Incomplete
❖ Complete
❖ Missed
❖ Septic

Induced
❖ Legal
❖ Illegal (criminal)

Threatened Abortion

It is a clinical entity where the process of abortion has started but has not progressed to a state from which recovery is impossible.

Clinical features:
1. Bleeding per vagina : The bleeding is usually slight and bright red in colour. On rare occasion, the bleeding may be brisk and sharp, specially in the second trimester, suggestive of low implantation of placenta. The bleeding usually stops spontaneously.
2. Pain: Usually painless, may be mild backache dull pain in lower abdomen. Pain appears usually following haemorrhage.

Inevitable Abortion

In this type of abortion where the changes have progressed to a state from where continuation of pregnancy is impossible.

Clinical Features:
1. Amenorrhoea
2. P/V bleeding
3. Lower abdominal pain : Aggravation of pain colicky in nature.
4. P/V examination /Bleeding Present (+)or (++) :
P/S: Dilated internal os of the cervix through which the products of   conception are felt.

Complete abortion

When product of conception are expelled completely.

Clinical Features:
1. Amenorrhoea
2. History of expulsion of fleshey mass per vagina.
3. Subsidence abdominal pain.
4. P/V bleeding: Trace or absent
5. P/V examination: Bleeding (+) or absent.

Bimanual examination:
1. Uterus is smaller than the period of amenorrhoea and firm.
2. Cervical os closed.
3. Bleeding: Trace or absent.

Incomplete abortion

When the entire products of conception are not expelled, instead a part of it is left inside the uterine cavity, it is called incomplete abortion. Commonest type of abortion amongst hospital incidence.

Clinical features:

1. Amenorrhoea

2. History of Expulsion of product of conception per vagina.

3. Continues lower abdominal colicky pain.

4. Per vaginal bleeding.(irregular).

5. Internal examination:

a. Uterus smaller than the period of amenorrhoea.

b. Patulous cervical os often admitting tip of the finger.

c. Varying amount of bleeding.(P/V)

Missed abortion

Sometimes fetus died in uterus and retained inside for a variable period is called missed abortion.

Clinical features:

1. Amenorrhoea

2. P/V bleeding / Brownish discharge.

3. Subsidence of pregnancy symptoms.

4. Fetal heart sound not audible with doppler.

5. Cervix feels firm.

6. Pregnancy test negative.

7. USG reveals absent fetal heart movement and fetal motion.

Complication: Blood coagulation disorders.

Recurrent (Habitual) Abortion

Three consecutive pregnancies ending in spontaneous abortion therefore constitute the criterion for the diagnosis of 'recurrent abortion'. In practice, however, investigation, if not treatment, may be justified by a woman's anxiety over having lost 2 pregnancies.

Criminal Abortion

Every women, being with child, who, with intent to procure her own miscarriage, shall unlawfully administer to herself any position or other noxious things.

Methods Used

1. Strong purgatives and single administrations of oxytocins.

2. Intra-uterine instrumentation: Domestic instruments such as hair pins, knitting needles and the like are frequently used.

3. Dilatation of the cervix

4. An intra-uterine injection

5. Potassium permanganate

Complications

a. Haemorrhage

b. Shock

c. Anuria

d. Peritonitis

e. Septicaemia

f.   Air embolism

g. Chemical embolism

h. Intravascular haemolysis

Diagnosis
Sings of recent injury to the
a. Cervix
b. Uterus
c. Vagina are found

Management
If the initial shock due to intravasation of solutions injected into the uterus does not respond to morphine, infusions, of blood and hydrocortisone given intravenously, exchange transfusion should be considered.
A. Removal of body of shock antibiotic evacuation of uterus.
B. Prevention.

Duty of a doctor in a case of criminal abortion:

❖ A criminal abortion is the induced destruction and expulsion of the foetus from the womb of the mother unlawfully when there is no therapeutic indication for the operation.

❖ The doctor's duty in this case is to guard all the informations obtained by him as a professional secrecy. He must urge the patient to make a statement about the induction of criminal miscarriage.

❖ If she refuses to make a statement, he should not pursue the matter. He must treat her to the best of his ability. He must consult a professional colleague.

❖ If the woman dies, he should not issue a death certificate, but should inform the police for making arrangement for postmortem examination.

❖ Under sec. 312 IPC whoever voluntarily causes criminal miscarriage is liable for imprisonment upto 3 years and or fine and if the woman is quick with the child the imprisonment mayextended upto 7 years.

❖ In this case, both the person procuring the miscarriage and the woman are liable for punishment. If this case, both the person procuring the miscarriage and the woman are liable for punishment.

❖ If the miscarriage is caused without the consent of the woman, the imprisonment may be upto 10 years under Sec.313 IPC.

❖ If the woman dies from the act of criminal abortions, the punishment is upto 10 years under sec.314 IPC, under sec.316 IPC causing death of quick unborn child by any act amounts to culpable homicide, and the punishment may extend upto 10 years of imprisonment.

REFERANCE
1. Basu S.C. , Hand Book Of Forensic Medicine and Toxicology, *third edition (2007),* Current Distributors, Lenin Saranee, Calcutta.
2. Mahanta Putul, Modern Textbook of Forensic Medicine And Toxicology *(2014),* Jaypee Brothers Medical Publishers, Darya Ganj, New Delhi.

3. Parikh C.K., Parikh's textbook of medical jurisprudence forensic medicine and toxicology, *sixth edition (2011),* C.B.S. Publishers and Distributors, Ansari Road, Darya Ganj, New Delhi.

4. Kumar Avinash, Law Of Evidence, *third edition (2011),* Singhal Law Publications, Burari, Delhi -84.

5. Modi. Jaising. P, Textbook of Medical Jurisprudence and Toxicology, Twenty *First Edition (1997),* N.M. Tripathi Private Limited, Bombay.

6. www.wikipedia.com

Chapter 20

VIRGINITY

VIRGINITY

Virginity

A female is called a virgin, if she never had any sexual intercourse and that state is called virginity.

MEDICOLEGAL IMPORTANCE

The question of virginity arises in following ways:-

- Comission of rape on a virgin woman
- Defamation: that a girl is not a virgin but a deflorated woman.
- Nullity of marriage and divorce

Marriage may be annulled that is declared never to have lawfully existed under the following conditions.

1. Where either party was already validly married with another subject and sings of loss of virginity are seen in the married female
2. Where the marriage has not been consummated due to impotence or willful refusal and the married woman remains virgin
3. Where the woman was not only deflorated but was also pregnant by another man at the time of marriage.

Other conditions of nullity of marriage other than loss of virginity are:

- ❖ When either party was under the age of marriage contract.
- ❖ Where the party was unsound mind or a mentally defective or suffering from communicable or curable diseases at the time of marriage.

SIGNS OF VIRGINITY[5]

GENITAL SINGS

1. **Labia majora:** Firm, elastic and rounded and lie in close contact with each other, even in full abduction of the thighs.
2. **Labia minora:** Soft and elastic, small and rose coloured. They lie in close contact and are not visible being hidden under the labia majora.
3. **Clitoris:** Not enlarged.
4. **Vestibule:** Narrow.
5. The posterior commissure and the fourchette are intact and crescent shaped.
6. **Vagina:** Narrow and tight with rugosed pinkish walls. Orifice is slit-like due to the presence of intact hymen.
7. **Perineum:** Entire or intact.
8. **Hymen;** An important sign of virginity is intact hymen but not the surest sign of virginity as in a female subject with elastic dilatable fimbriated and fleshy hymen remains intact even after sexual intercourse.
9. Uterus is very small and not palpable with signs of nulliparous uterus.

EXTRA GENITAL SINGS

1. Breast is hemispherical, firm, plump and elastic.
2. Nipple is small and pointed, surrounded by pink colour small areola.
3. Abdomen show no signs of enlargement, recent or old other signs due to pregnancy.

Hymen: a thin membrane that surrounds the opening to the vagina. Hymens can come in different shapes. The most common hymen in young girls is shaped like a half moon. This shape allows menstrual blood to flow out of a girl's vagina.

Types of Hymens

1. **Imperforate hymen**: An imperforate hymen can be diagnosed at birth. Rarely, the diagnosis isn't made until the teen years. An imperforate hymen is a thin membrane that completely covers the opening to the vagina. Menstrual blood cannot flow out of the vagina. This usually causes the blood to back up into the vagina which often develops into an abdominal mass and abdominal and/or back pain. Some teens may also have pain with bowel movements and difficulty passing urine.

2. The treatment for an imperforate hymen is minor surgery to remove the extra hymenal tissue and create a normal sized vaginal opening so that menstrual blood can flow out of the vagina.

3. **Microperforate hymen**: A microperforate hymen is a thin membrane that almost completely covers the opening to a young women's vagina. Menstrual blood is usually able to flow out of the vagina but the opening is very small. A teen with a microperforate hymen usually will not be able to get a tampon into her vagina and may not realize that she has a very tiny opening. If she is able to put a tampon into her vagina she may not be able to remove it when it becomes filled with blood. The treatment is minor surgery to remove the extra hymenal tissue making a normal sized opening for menstrual blood to flow out.

4. **Septate hymen**: A septate hymen is when the thin hymenal membrane has a band of extra tissue in the middle that causes two small vaginal openings instead of one. Teens with a septate hymen may have trouble getting a tampon in or trouble getting a tampon out. The treatment for a septate hymen is minor surgery to remove the extra band of tissue and create a normal sized vaginal opening.

Various Types of Hymens

Annular hymen
Septate hymen
Cribriform hymen

Imperforate hymen
Parous introitus (after childbirth)

Definitions of virginity loss

There are varying understandings as to which types of sexual activities result in loss of virginity. The traditional view is that virginity is only lost through vaginal penetration by the penis, consensual or non-consensual, and that acts of oral sex, anal sex and mutual masturbation do not result in loss of virginity. A person who engages in such acts with no history of having engaged in vaginal intercourse is often regarded among heterosexuals and researchers as "technically a virgin". In contrast, gay or lesbian individuals may describe such acts as resulting in loss of virginity. Some gay males regard anal penetration as resulting in loss of virginity, but not oral sex, and lesbians may regard oral sex or fingering as loss of virginity. Some lesbians debate the traditional definition and whether or not non-penile forms of vaginal penetration constitute virginity loss, while other gays and lesbians assert that the term "virginity" is useless to them because of the prevalence of the traditional definition.[5]

CHANGES IN HYMEN AFTER RUPTURE

- The ruptured portion portion hymen looks like triangular projections varying from 3-6 in number in 5'o clock and 7'o clock position usually.

- The tear will usually reach upto the base that is vaginal attachment torn site shows evidence of inflammation, tender to touch with signs of healing.it heals up from edges by 4-6 days,but torn segment will never reunite.

- After rupture the segments gradually become thicker and smaller in size and are revealed as small fleshy pyramidal projections, which are known as corunculae hymenalis or myritiformis: they disappear only after the child birth or after repeated sexual intercourse extending over a long period.

MEDICOLEGAL ASPECT

- ❖ There is no single sign which can be called surest sign of virginity or absolute sign of defloration. The presence of unruptured hymen affords presumptions, but is not an absolute proof of virginity. The diagnosis of virginity and defloration is difficult and in many cases a physical examination of the genital organs only may not be helpful.
- ❖ With an intact elastic hymen there are false virgins; there are causes of rupture of hymen other than sexual intercourse.
- ❖ The hymen is present always in a virgin in some form or other than sexual intercourse.
- ❖ The hymen is present always in a virgin in some form or other, but very rarely may be absent congenitally.

References

1. C.K Parikh, Parikh's textbook of medical jurisprudence, forensic medicine and toxicology, 6th e P.5.1,5.3,5.5,5.6,5.8,5.10,5.11,5.12
2. A.K Gupta, Essentials of forensic medicine and toxicology, P.150-155
3. www.forensicindia.com/ugteaching/forensictoxicology.pdf, Imran Sabri
4. Wikipedia.org/wiki/forensictoxicology

5. Krishan Vij Textbook of Forensic medicine and Toxicology, 4th Edt.

Chapter 21

DELIVERY

DELIVERY

The cases in which the medical jurist is required to ascertain whether a woman has been delivered or not are those of abortion, infanticide , concealment of birth, feigned delivery, contested legitimacy, libel action of disrupted chastity, and blackmail.[1]

Delivery means the expulsion or extraction of the child at birth. Sometimes, a doctor is asked to examine a woman for signs of delivery and, if there is evidence of such delivery, to state the probable time since her delivery. While there is no general diagnostic sign, the sign of delivery are better marked, the more recent the delivery and the more mature the child. Hence, it is important to make the examination at the earliest possible moment.[2]

Stages of Labour:

Stages of labour are divided into three stages:

i.   **First stage:** it starts from the onset of true labour pain and ends with full dialatation of the cervix. It is cervical stage of labour. Its average duration is 12 hours in primigravidae and 6 hours in multiparae.

ii.   **Second stage:** it starts with the full dialatation of the cervix not from the rupture of the membranes) and ends with expulsion of the fetus from the birth canal. It has got two phases-

iii. **(a) Propulsive phase**: starts from full dialatation upto the descent of the presenting part to the pelvic floor.

    (b) Expulsive phase: is distinguished by maternal bearing down efforts and ends with delivery of the baby. Its average duration is 2 hours in primigravidae and 30 minutes in multiparae.

iv.   **Third stage:** it begins after expulsion of the fetus and ends with the expulsion of the placenta and membranes after birth. The average duration is about 15 minutes in both primigravidae and multiparae.[5]

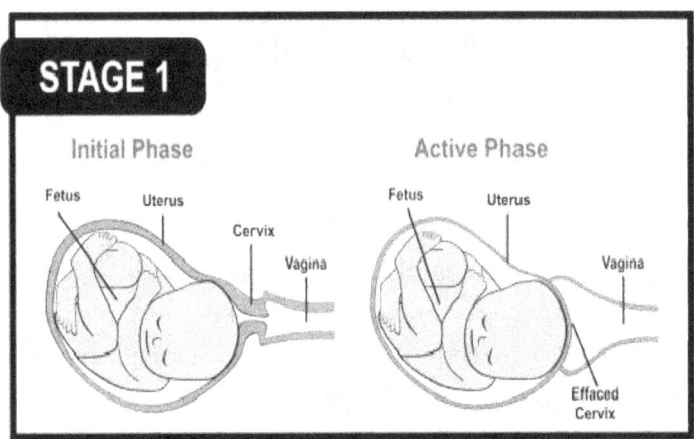

STAGE 1

Initial Phase   Active Phase

Fetus   Uterus   Fetus   Uterus

Cervix   Vagina

Vagina

Effaced
Cervix

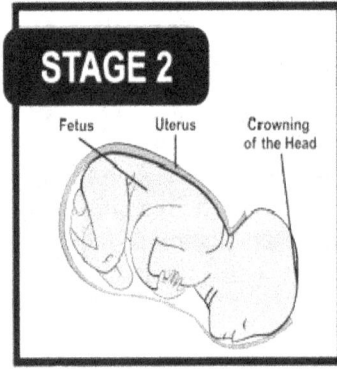

STAGE 2

Fetus   Uterus   Crowning
of the Head

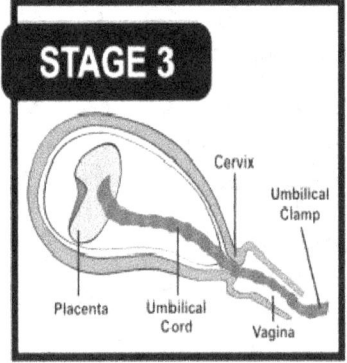

STAGE 3

Cervix

Umbilical
Clamp

Placenta   Umbilical
Cord   Vagina

EVENTS IN FIRST STAGE OF LABOUR

The first stage is chiefly concerned with the preparation of birth canal so as to facilitate expulsion of fetus in the second stage. The main events that occur in first stage are:

Dilatation of cervix: softening of the cervix, fibro-musculo-glandular hypertrophy, increased vascularity, accumulation of fluid in between collagen fibres and breaking down of collagen fibrils by enzymes collagenase and elastate.

Cervical Effacement and Dilatation During Labor

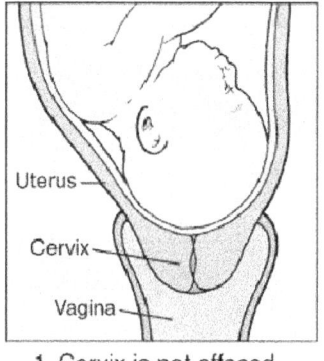

1. Cervix is not effaced or dilated.

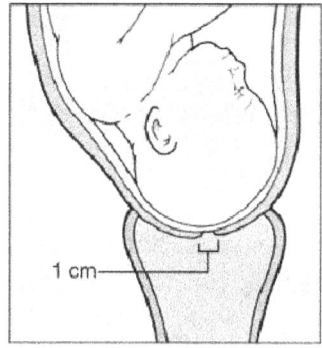

2. Cervix is fully effaced and dilated to 1 cm.

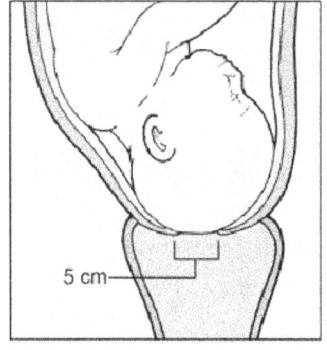

3. Cervix is dilated to 5 cm.

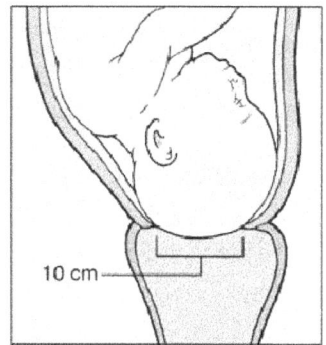

4. Cervix is fully dilated to 10 cm.

Uterine contraction and retraction

Bag of membranes: the membranes (amnion and chorion) are attached loosely to the deciduas lining the uterine cavity except over the internal os. The amniotic fluid is divided into two compartments. The part above the girdle of contact contains the fetus with bulk of liquor is known as hindwaters and the one below it containing small amount of liquor is called forewaters.

Fetal axis pressure.

Effacement or taking up of cervix.

Full formation of Lower uterine segment.[5]

EVENTS IN SECOND STAGE OF LABOUR

This stage is concerned with the descent and delivery of the fetus trough the birth canal.

Second stage has two phases:

A. Propulsive: from full dilatation until head touches the pelvic floor.

B. Expulsive: since the time mother has irresistible desire to 'bear down' and push until the baby is delivered.[5]

EVENTS IN THIRD STAGE OF LABOUR

The third stage of labour comprises the phase of placental separation; its descent to the lower segment and finally its expulsion with the membranes.[5]

Placental separation

There are two ways of placental separation:

1) Central separation (schultze): detachment of placenta from its uterine attachment starts at the centre resulting in opening up of few uterine sinuses and accumulation of blood behind the placenta. With increasing contraction, more and more detachment occurs until whole of the placenta gets detached.

2) Marginal separation (Mathews-Duncan): separation starts at the margin as it is mostly unsupported. With progressive uterine contraction, more and more ares of placenta gets deatached. It is found more frequently. [5]

Expulsion of placenta

After complete separation of the placenta, it is forced down into the flabby lower uterine segment or upper part of the vagina by effective contraction and retraction of the uterus. Thereafter, it is expelled out by either voluntary contraction of abdominal muscles or by manual procedure.[5]

SIGNS OF DELIVERY

These signs are discussed under the following four headings:-

- ❖ Signs of recent delivery in the living.
- ❖ Signs of recent delivery in the dead.
- ❖ Signs of remote delivery in the living.
- ❖ Signs of remote delivery in the dead.[1,2,3]

SIGNS OF RECENT DELIVERY IN THE LIVING

The signs of recent delivery at full term are:-

1. Appearance of general indisposition-For the first 2 or 3 days after delivery the woman wears a languished look with the sunken eyes having a dusky pigmentation about the lower eyelids, and has a slight increase in the pulse and temperature. These signs may be absent in strong woman, or may be found in any other illness or at the time of the monthly course. The intermittent contractions of the uterus are usually present for the first 4 or 5 days. These are termed after pains when they are vigorous and painful.

2. Breast: The breasts are full, firm, knotty and enlarged, and contain colostrums or milk. The areolae are dark, Montgomery's glandular tubercles are seen, superficial veins are prominent and the nipples are turgid.

3. Abdomen: The abdomen is slightly full, but more often lax and flabby. The skin is wrinkled and shows the lineae-albicantes, which are pinkish in the beginning, but subsequently become white in colour.

4. Uterus: Just after delivery the uterus relaxes and may be felt as a flabby mass extending to the umbilicus a few hours after delivery. It then diminishes in size about 1 cm. a day , and is felt like a hard cricket ball for about two or three days in the lower part of the abdomen above the symphysis pubis, but its fundus can be felt just above or behind the symphysis pubis up to the fourteenth day.

5. Vagina: The labia are tender swollen gaping and bruised or lacerated. The vagina is smooth relaxed and dilated, and may show recenttears, which usually heal by seventh day. The fourchette is usually ruptured, and perineum is sometimes lacerated.

6. Cervix: The cervix is soft and patulous, and its edges are torn or lacerated transversely. The internal os begins to close during the first 24 hours. The external os is soft and patent admitting 2 fingers for a few days. It admits with difficulty 1 finger at the end of a week, and closes in 2 weeks.

7. Lochia: This is a discharge from the uterus and vagina, it has a peculiar, sour, disagreeable odour. During the first 4 to 5 days the discharge is bright red (lochia rubra) consisting of pure blood mixed with large clots and is strongly suggestive of recent delivery. It becomes serous and paler in colour (lochia serosa) during the next four days. About the ninth day the colour becomes yellowish, gray or slightly greenish (lochia alba or green water), and gradually diminishes in quantity, till it disappears altogether in about 2 weeks.[1,2]

Types

a) Lochia rubra (1-4 days) is bright red in colour and consists of blood, shreds of fetal membranes and deciduas, vernixcaseosa, lanugo and meconium.

b) Lochia serosa (5-9 days) is watery and pale and consist of less RBC but more leukocyte, wound , exudates, mucus from the cervix and microorganism (anaerobic streptococci and staphylococci).

c) Lochia alba (10-15 days) is scanty, thicker, greyish, yellow and then whitish till final disappearance it contains decidual cells, leukocytes, mucous, cholesterol crystal, fatty and granular epithelial cells and microorganism.

Significance of lochia

The average amount of discharge for first 4-5 days is about 250 ml. if it smells offensive, then it indicates infection. If scanty or absent or excessive infection; persistence of red colour beyond normal subinvolution or retain bits of conceptus; and duration beyond 3 weeks suggest local genital lesions.4

LABORATORY INVESTIGATIONS
Immunological tests are positive for about 7-10 days after delivery.
From the above signs taken collectively it will scarcely be difficult to diagnose a case of recent delivery for the first fourteen days after parturition. These signs are more characteristic of a full –term delivery than of a premature one. They are likely to disappear within a week, or ten days or even at an earlier date in a strong and vigorous woman, especially if she happens to be a multipara.[1,2]
The examination for evidence of recent delivery should include an examination for any sign which would be consistent with a precipitate labour.

If it is the first child, general appearance of indisposition may be present. The woman may look pale, exhausted and ill. The pulse is soft and quick and there is a slight increase in temperature. The intermittent concentrations of the uterus, known as after-pains, are usually present for the first four or five days. These signs are not diagnostic for recent delevery as they may be found in any other illness or at the time of the monthly course. The signs of general indisposition may be absent in strong women.

Besides the general appearance, breasts are enlarged, tense and knotty. The surface veins are dilated and there is dark pigmentation round the nipples. Striae are seen on the breasts and Montgomery's tubercles are found. On pressure, colostrum can be squeezed out for about ten days after delivery. It is replaced by milk thereafter.

The abdomen is lax and shows striaegravidarum and lineanigra. The diagnosis does not depend on the external appearances mentioned here but on the local examination.

The vulva is bruised and gaping, the vagina is roomy, the fourchette and posterior commisure and destroyed, and the perineum may be lacetrated, the age of the tear being of value to fix the date of delivery. The uterus is enlarged. It does not shrink to its original size immediately after delivery. The fundus lies about two and one-half centimeters below the umbilicus. It diminishes at the rate of about one and one-half centimeters a day for the first few day. On palpation, it feels like a hard cricket ball for about two or three days, in the lower abdomen above the pubis. By the tenth day, it is on level with brim if the pelvis. In from two or three weeks, the fundus sinks below the level of the pubis into the pelvic cavity. It reaches its normal size in about six weeks. The cervix is soft and patulous and its edges torn and lacerated transversely. The internal os begins to close within the first twenty four hours, the external os is soft and patent admitting two fingers for the first few days, and one finger with difficulty at the end of a week. It closes in two weeks. There is caginal discharge, with a peculiar sour disagreeable odour. This discharge is known as lochia. It contains red cells, leucocytes, decidual debris, vaginal epithilium, peptones, and cholesterol crystals. During the first three days, it is blood stained and therefore known as lochia rubra. During the next three day, it becomes paler serous and therefore known as lochia serosa. After the next three days it becomes yellowish or greenish and then whitish, when it is known as lochia alba. It then gradually loses all colour till it finally disappears in about fifteen days. Lochia is discharge which is the part of the healing process of the uterus after delivery. The discharge is therefore blood stained in the beginning and whitish later. All the above signs are more characteristic of a full term delivery then of a premature one. They are likely to dissappear within about ten days or even earlier in a strong and vigorous women especially if she happens to be multipara.

From the extent of stretching and laceration of the part, an idea may be obtained of the size of the foetus, or if this is known, the rapidity of the birth may be guaged. The sooner a women is examined after an alleged delivery, the greater are the chances of obtaining useful information. The biological tests may be of value in certain cases. They remain positive for about a week or so after delivery. Usually, after two or three weeks, it is impossible to fix the date of delivery with degree ofcertainty[3].

Signs of recent delivery (both living and dead)

- ❖ Engorged breasts
- ❖ Pink striae on the abdomen
- ❖ Enlarged uterus
- ❖ Fresh tears of the vulva, vagina or cervix
- ❖ Lochia from the uterus[4]

Signs of Remote Delivery in the Living

A previous pregnancy usually leaves permanent marks on a woman especially if the pregnancy has gone to full term the extent and characters of the signs found will depend upon whether the women is primiparous or multiparous. The diagnosis of a previous pregnancy may be considered justifiable if all or a majority of the following signs are present.

The breasts are lax, soft and pendulous. They are frequently wrinkled if the woman nursed her baby occasionally show subcutaneous scars [lineaalbicantes]. The nipples are enlarged with a persistent dark areola around them, and montgomery's tubercles are usually present. Milk can frequently be squeezed from the nipples. The abdominal walls tend to be lax and show the presence of lines albicantes on the lateral aspects. There is commonly a deeply pigmented line [lineanigra] from the pubis to the umbilicus. There may be a scar due to old laceration of the perineum and the absence of signs virginity, that is, the hymen is ruptured, the vagina open and gaping, and a non-rugose condition of the vaginal walls. These signs do not prove that delivery has taken place as they may be simulated by other conditions, and if only one child has been born, these signs may be very slight. The only sign which proves delivery is the appearance of the os uteri in a parous woman, the internal os is not well defined while the external os is transverse, irregular, fissured, and may admit the tip of the finger. In a nulliparous woman, the internal os is well defined while the external os is rounded with a dimple in the centre and the orifice.[1,2,4]

Signs of Remote delivery in the dead

The uterus is larger, thicker and heavier than the nulliparuos uterus. However, it must be remembered that uterus undergose atrophy in old age. The walls are concave from inside forming a wider and rounded cavity, while the walls of the nulliparous uterus are convex on the inner aspect and from savity which is smaller in capicity and triangular in shape. The top of the fundus in a parous woman is convex and on a higher level than that of the broad ligaments; in a nulliparous woman, it is at level with the broad ligaments. The cervix and the body are about the same length in the virgin, while in a parous woman, the body is twice the length of the cervix and in the later, the arbor vitae have disapeared. Arbor vitae is the name given to the mucosal folds in the canal of uterine cervix which extends from internal so to external os. The canal is spindle shaped and has two transverse. Mucosal folds, one on anterior and another on posterior edge of the canal. Numerous oblique mucosal folds run from these transverse folds, giving the appearance of a tree and hence the name arbor vitae. The edges of the cervix may show cicatrices on account of previous tears and lacerations caused during delivery. The external os is enlarged and the internal os is not so well defined as that in the virgin. The placental site is elevated and tinged with blood pigment for six months, and on cutting sections, enderteritisobliterans can be seen in the blood vessels for years afterwards.

Medicolegal aspect[1,2]

Medcolegal importance of devielivery comes up in connection with the following-

- ❖ Avoiding court attendance by the pregnant woman for giving evidence on the ground of illness following delivery.
- ❖ Prayer for changing death sentence to life imprisonment on the ground of delivery and rearing up the infant.
- ❖ Legitimacy.
- ❖ Libel action for disputed chastity of a woman.
- ❖ Feigned delivery.
- ❖ Charged for commiting abortion and infanticide.
- ❖ Concealment of birth of infant after home delivery.

❖ Blackmailing a woman.

Signs of recent delivery

In a living subject:

Extragenital signs

1. A general appearence of indisposition (commonly seen in primigravida)

    a) Languished look (exhausted facis).
    b) Sunken eyes.
    c) Dusky pigmentation of lower eyelids.
    d) Slight increases of pulse rate and temperature.

But these signs may be found in cases of woman suffering from severe illness, while they may be absent in cases of-

(a) Woman having severe children, and

(b) Very strong woman.

2. Heavy puerperal odour around her body.

3. Breast- full, firm, knotty, enlarged with prominent superfical veins. Colostrum and milk comes out of nipple. Areola is dark and the nipple is turgid.

4. Abdomen shows slight fullness, but more often lax and flabby. The skin is wrikled and shows linea-albicantes (straegravidarum) which are pink at the begining, but later becomes white.

Signs in genital organs

1. **Uterus-** Just after the delivery the uterus relaxes and may be felt as flabby muscular tumour like mass extending to the umbilicus in size; it is felt as hard cricket ball for about 2-3 days in lower part of the abdomen 3 cm below umbilicus and a little above the symphysis pubis. The intermittent contractions of the uterus are usually palpable upto 4-5 days after delivery. Vigorous contractions may lead to after-pain. Peritoneum covering lower part of uterus folds for 2-3 days after delivery. Uterus usually diminishes in size at the rate 1.5 cm per day.

2. In a case of normal delivery cervix is soft, patulous, edges of external os are torn or lacerated transversely. Internal os begins to close within 24 hours.

External os is soft and patent admitting two fingers for a few days after delivery. It admits 1 finger tightly at the end of a week and closes in 2 weeks. In case of multipara, external, os is a transverse slit or torn at the edge; this is the most important finding as in case of nulliparous as woman external is round with a dimple at the centre.

3. Vagina is smooth relaxed and dilated and may show recent tears.

4. Vulva is swollen, may be bruised and lacerated.

5. Fourchette and perineum may show tears and lacerations. Episiotomy with stiching is seen in primigrarida.

6. Lochical discharge from the uterus coming out from vagina is the characteristics sign of all recent deliveries. It presents a peculiar, sour disagreeable (peurperal) odour.

During the first 3-4 days bright red discharge consisting of blood mixed with large clots come out from uterus. During next 4 days it is serous and paler. At about the 9th day, it becomes yellowish grey or may be slightly pale greenish and disappears altogether from 2nd or 3rd week after delivery. It may persist upto 4th week

according to constitution of the patient.[4]

In a dead subject

In addition to the findings mentioned in living female: Subjects, post-mortem examination reveal following sings:

1. The enlarged flabby uterus can be seen after opening the abdomen. Wrinkling of the peritoneal covering over it may be seen.

2. When the uterus is cut open the dark coloured placental site will be seen, showing opened up placental sinus. Placental site appears as an irregular elevated area about 12-15 cm in diameter and covered with clotted blood. The site measure 3-4 cm at the end of first week.

3. In recent cases, ovaries and fallopian tubes will be found congested and corpus luteum will be found in the ovaries.

4. Changes in uterus after delivery helps to opine how many hours and days

after delivery the pregnant female died:

(i) After full term recent delivery uterus is about 20-25 cm in diameter externally and 15-18 cm internally and weighs nearly about 1000 gms.

(ii) After 2-3 days it is about 17 cm long, 10 cm broad and weights about 500 gms. (iii) At the end of a week it is about 12.5 cm in lenghts, 2.5 cm thick and weights roughly 350 gms.

(iv) After 15 days it is 10-12 cm long and weights roughly 170 gms.

(v) Almost normal pre-parous size is attained by 6 weeks when it measures 9 cmX 6.5 cmX 2.5 cm (weight 80-120 gms).

(vi) 14-21 days after delivery the uterus may become retroverted in position.

5. Urinary bladder may show extensive congestion and may contain blood mixed urine specially in difficult recent delivery.

Signs of remote delivery

In a living subjects

A. Extragenital signs:

1. Abdomen- Lax and marks of lineaalbicantes are seen on front and sides of abdomen lower uterine caesarean section (LUCS) linear old surgical scar on front of abdomen, a little above symphsis pubis may be seen.

2. Breast are enlarged pendulous, lax and tender, especially after several deliveries. Nipples are prominent and blunt with dark areola around them.

B. Genital signs:

3. Labias: Labia majora and especially the minora are separated apart.

4. Vaginal canal is patulous, orifice gaping and its mucosa does not show any rugae.

5. Perineum shows evidence of old healed rupture in some cases.

6. Cervix is irregular enlarged.

7. External os is seen as transverse slit-like opening and may be patulous. However, many of these signs may be absent in a woman, who had a delivery before the full term or had a caesarean section. It is possible for the vagina and vulva to regain the near non-pregnant state in such case.

In a dead subject

In a addition to above findings in living female subjects post-mortem examination reveal following signs:

1. Uterus is slightly enlarged, cavity larger, walls thickened and weights is greater than nulliparous uterus. Placental site measure 1-2 cm in diameter six weeks after delivery. Placental site is recognisable even up to 12 weeks after delivery.

2. External os- slit like opening but not patulous.[3]

Written informed consent needs to be taken before examination after explaining reasons and possible consequencies[4.]

Size of uterus after delivery

Time after delivery	Dimension(cm)	Weight(g)	Placental site diameter
Immediate	20 X 15 X5	1000	10-15
1st week	14 X 8 X 4	500	4
2nd week	12 X 7 X 3	300	2.5
3rd week	9 X 5 X 3	100	1.5

Referance

1. Modi. Jaising. P, Textbook of Medical Jurisprudence And Toxicology, Twenty *First Edition (1997),* N.M. Tripathi Private Limited, Bombay.
2. Parikh C.K., Parikh's textbook of medical jurisprudence forensic medicine and toxicology, *sixth edition (2011),*C.B.S. Publishers and Distributors, Ansari Road, Darya Ganj, New Delhi.
3. A.K Gupta, Essential of Forensic Medicine and Toxicology, Fifth Edition, The Indian Press Pvt Ltd, 93A Lenin Saranee, Kolkata.
4. Mahanta Putul, Modern Textbook of Forensic Medicine And Toxicology *(2014),* Jaypee Brothers Medical Publishers, Darya Ganj, New Delhi. .
5. Konar Hirala, Textbook of obstetrics, seventh edition (2013), New central book agency, Kolkata.
6. Wikipedia

Chapter 22

LEGITIMACY

LEGITIMACY

It is the legal state of a person born in lawful wedlock [1-5].

LEGITIMATE CHILD

Under section 112 of the Indian Evidence Act, a legitimate child has been defined s one born during the continuance of a valid marriage between his mother and any man or within 280 days after its dissolution of divorce, or death of the husband, and the mother remaining unmarried.[1,3,4,5]

ILLEGITIMATE CHILD

An illegitimate or bastard child is one which is born out of wedlock or not within a competent time after the cessation of the relationship of man and wife or born within wedlock when procreation by the husband is not possible, because of congenital or acquired malformation or illness.[4]

The child becomes illegitimate or bastard, if it can be proved that the husband could not possibly be the father of the child in following circumstances:-

(i)   The alleged father has not attained the age of puberty.

(ii)   He is physically incapable of performing sexual intercourse or cannot deposit semen in vagina of his wife because of illness or congenital or acquired deformities.

(iii)   He did not have sexual access to his wife when the child was begotten (i.e. not born out of legal wedlock).

(iv)   The blood group and DNA pattern of the child and the alleged father are not compatible (see Chapter on Blood groups).[1-3,5]

AN ILLEGITIMATE CHILD BECOMES LEGITIMATE BY THE SUBSEQUENT MARRIAGE OF PARENTS IF THE CHILD IS BORN OUT OF LAWFUL WEDLOCK.[1]

WHEN QUESTION OF LEGITIMACY ARISES?

The question of legitimacy and disputed paternity arises under the following circumstances, viz.

    (1)   Nullity of marriage

    (2)   Divorce

    (3)   Inheritance

    (4)   Affiliation (adoption) cases, and

    (5)   Suppositious children.

- **Nullity of Marriage:** Legally, marriage is a contract and it can be nullified if

  (a) Either party is under the age of marriage contract

  (b) Either party was already validity married.

  (c) Both parties are of the same sex

  (d) Either party was suffering from incurable impotency, insanity, HIV infection, leprosy, or venereal disease in a communicable form prior to marriage

  (e) Either party was so intoxicated at the time of marriage as not to understand the nature of the marriage contract

  (f) There is wilful refusal to consummate marriage, and

  (g) The respondent wife at the time of marriage was pregnant by any person other than the husband.

- **Divorce:** This means dissolution of a previously valid marriage. If the intrauterine age of the child is proved to be greater than the period of access between the parents, the dissolution of marriage is allowed by the court on the grand of adultery. The other grounds for divorce include:

  (a) desertion

  (b) cruelty

  (c) criminal sex practices, e.g. rape, sodomy, or bestiality and incurable sanity

(d) HIV infection

(e) Leprosy or venereal disease in a communicable form.[1]

- **Inheritance:** Inheritance of property etc. by a posthumous child. (Posthumous child is a child born after the death of his father, and the mother must have conceived by the said father. It is a legitimate child and it can inherit the property left by its father).[2]

A legitimate child born during lawful wedlock can inherit the property of its father.[4,5]

Only a legitimate child can inherit property of its parents. Hence, in a case of inheritance, the question of legitimacy of a child may arise and medical evidence may be required concerning the following facts, viz.

(1) Age in regard to pregnancy

(2) Duration of pregnancy

(3) Unusual forms of pregnancy, such, as super fecundation and superfoetation,

(4) Paternity.

- **AGE IN REGARD TO PREGNANCY:** While from time to time cases are recorded of young girls delivering children, in India, at present eighteen years is the earliest age at which a female can contract a valid marriage and a legitimate conception can take place. Greater importance is probably associated with the age of certain women at the time of their delivery late in life, since important legal issues may emerge.

- **DURATION OF PREGNANCY:** While the normal average duration of pregnancy is accepted as 280 days which is equal to fen times the normal intermenstrual period of 28 days, it must be considered possible that the duration of pregnancy could be shorter or loner where the individual menstrual cycle is a shorter or longer.

Where the duration of gestation is shorter than normal, the question of viability of child arises. Viability means the stage of maturity at which a foetus with normal intrauterine development is able to maintain a separate existence after birth. A child is viable after 210 days or seven months of intrauterine life, or rarely 180 days or six months but in most of these cases the foetus is immature. The stage of maturity is generally reflected by the weight of the child at birth.

A four pound baby was born after a gestation period of 173 says. On medical evidence that the baby was normal and survived normally without any special care of efforts to keep it alive, the Court accepted the husband's contention that he was not the father of the child and granted divorce. (Bombay High Court First Appeal No. 666 of 1959).

Where the duration of gestation if longer than normal, the child must be larger and heavier than normal, and the ossific centres more fully developed, or else it is unusual and suspicious. Mckeown and Gibson from their investigation on 15.628 births conclude that for medicolegal purposes, a period of 354 days from coitus to birth is not impossible (BMJ: 1952, 1, 938-941).

- **Unusual forms of pregnancy: Superfecundation and Superfoetation are unusual forms of pregnancy**

(a) Superfecundation

By superfecundation is meant the fertilization of two ova of the same period of ovulation by two separate acts of coitus committed at short internals. This occurrence is possible, but it is difficult to prove in human beings, since both fertilized ova develop as twins and go to full term at about the same periods. A law suit[23] about the paternity of twins is reported, where it was contended on the basis of blood group tests that the defendant could not have been the father of one of the twins, that is, the twins must have had two father, and this in turn, would prove the possibility of superfecundation in human beings.[4]

The incidence of twin pregnancies of about 1-1.5% (1 in 80) and, of those, binovular twins resulting from separate fertilisation of two ova formed the same menstrual cycle are 5-6 times more common than uniovular twins. Both the zygote do not always develop to maturity One foetus may die and be retained until the labour that expels the other. The dead foetus may be flattened by pressure and may be unrecognisable and is referred to as a foetus compressus or foetus papyraceus. The spermatozoa, causing fertilisation may be from different men. The rare case where two ova of same cycle are fertilised by a white and black person with entirely different blood groups are the unique example of this condition.[2]

A case has been recorded in literature where a woman who had coitus first with a fait-skinned male and subsequently with a dark-skinned male gave birth to twins one of which was fair-skinned and the other dark-skinned and both equally developed.

Herberer records a case of disputed paternity where on the basis of blood group tests, it was contended that the defendant could not have been the father of one of the twins.[1]

(b) Superfoetation

By Superfoetation is meant the fertilisation of two separate ova discharged from the ovary at different period of ovulation. Since menstruation may take place for two or three months after impregnation has occurred, superfoetation is possible during this period, but is must be regarded as a very unlikely occurrence. It may occur in cases of double uterus or uterus didelphis. Two infants in different stages of development may be born.

It is the impregnation of another ovum belonging to subsequent period of ovulation after the ovum discharged from a previous ovulation has already been developing as a foetus for a month or more. This is not possible after 3 months of pregnancy as the decidua vera comes into apposition with the decidua reflexa and thus the decidual cavity is obliterated and uterine end of fallopian tube are blocked.

Here, two foetuses are born either at the same time showing different stages of development or two fully developed foetuses are born at different periods varying from 1 to 3 months later to former.

Some experts deny possibility of this condition. Cases where a second fully developed child was born explained time after the first, have been explained on the assumption of twin pregnancy in which the second child did not develop ether due to diminished blood supply or some other cause. On the birth of the normally developed child, the second foetus received proper nourishment and is subsequently born as mature child. However, superfoetation may not only be a possibility but a reality in a bipartite or double uterus.

The following case recorded by Tyler Smith conclusively proves the occurrence of superfoetation:

- A young married woman, pregnant for the first time, miscarried at the end of the fifth month, and some hours afterwards a small clot was discharged enclosing a perfectly healthy had menstruated regularly during the period that she had been pregnant.

- John M. Murray reports that the post mortem examination on the body of a coloured woman, aged 35 years, who died from pulmonary tuberculosis, the uterus contained a well-formed foetus of thirteen or fourteen weeks, and a much smaller embryo of six weeks was found in the left Fallopian tube.

- Sussi also reports a case superfoetation. A primipara aged 32, gave birth to a full term boy and twenty minutes later to a living female foetus of about sixth foeta month. There was a great different in the sizes and in weights of the foetuses, the ratio being 7:1 and there was also a considerable difference in the two placentas.

- A case is mentioned in which female labourer from Mangalore gave birth to a child on December 22, 1948, and after an interval of 18 days she was delivered of another child. The lady doctor who attended her stated that this was due to the fact the woman had a double uterus.

- Bhagwat describes a case of a seven para woman, who gave birth to a child in the seventh month of the pregnancy. The child died on the second day. After about twenty six days she was delivered from the hospital. On examination, it was found that this was result of a bicornuate uterus. All the other deliveries were normal.

- Cases of supposed superfoetation may, however, be explained in other ways. If twins are born together of apparently very unequal development, this may be due to simply to one of the twins having failed to obtain an equal share of nutriment during intra-uterine life. If the less developed foetus is not alive, it is almost certain that is simply a case of blighted ovum retained without decomposition.

Paternity: The word paternity literally means fatherhood but the term is used here in a broader sense to mean parenthood. The supposes parent may or may not be real father. In cases of disputed paternity, blood group tests are resorted to in India, these tests are carried out by the Haffkine Institute in Bombay, Central Forensic Science Laboratory at Delhi, the Serologist of India at Calcutta, and several other Forensic Science Laboratories all over the Country. DNA testing is not yet common.

Paternity of a child may have to be determined in case of illegitimacy. This is usually done by detailed blood grouping tests and taking into account the resemblance of the child's feature with the said father, DNA study may be necessary for final setting of this dispute.

(a) **Parental likeness** – The child may resemble the father in feature and figure and other personal peculiarities which characterise the alleged father. Such evidences are regarded merely as corroborative ones.'

(b) **Atavism-** Here the child does not resemble its parents, but resembles its grand-parents. This is due to inheritance of characteristics from remote rather than from immediate ancestors, possibly due to a chance recombination of genes.

(c) **Blood group tests used in paternity determination –** The elaborate study of the blood group of the alleged parents and the child may provide evidence about the possibility of a certain person being the father of the child, or when two persons are involved, in deciding which of the two male could be father of the child.

(d) D.N.A. test are done now a days for fixation of paternity and maternity of the child.

The possibility of mutation is very important in paternity exclusion tests. Mutation is a change in gene between generations resulting in an altered character in the child. The possible risk of error in paternity determination by blood grouping due to mutation has been estimated by Race and Sanger as not more than 1 in 50,000.

Affiliation (Adoption) cases: These are popularly known as suits for adoption. They are cases which are brought before the court for fixing the paternity of an illegitimate child. Under section 125 CrPC, an individual must adopt his illegitimate child or support him up to a certain age. In the latter case, a magistrate of the first class may make a maximum allowance of rupees 500 hundred per month for the maintenance of such a child, after taking into consideration only the necessities of life, such as food, clothing and lodging and not luxury.[1,2]

A woman may allege a particular man to be the father of her child and file a case in the court for fixing the paternity. If this paternity is fixed on a certain person, he becomes responsible to support the child. Blood grouping and DNA analysis can prove the allegation[3,5].

These are the case which are brought before court for fixing the paternity of an illegitimate child upon a certain individual as he is bound, under section 125 of the Indian Criminal Procedure Code, to support his legitimate child which is unable to maintain itself irrespective of age.[3] In such cases blood grouping tests may be necessary but in India under the present law it is held that the courts are not empowered to direct that such tests to be made, when the proceedings are in quasi civil matters.[4] In England the Court of appeal recently decided that the High Court had power to order a child's blood to be tested in paternity issues (The times, May 28, 1968).[4a] A Magistrate of the first class may make a monthly allowance of any sum not exceeding five hundred rupees on the whole for the maintenance of such child. In determining the amount of maintenance, luxury is not to be taken into consideration but only the necessaries of life viz. food, clothing and lodgiong[4].

Suppositious Children: A suppositious child means a fictitious child. A woman may pretend pregnancy s well as delivery and later produce a child as if it is her own. She may substitute a living male child for a dead child or for a living female child born of her. The purpose is to extort money by blackmail or divert succession to property. The medical office must be able to say from the examination of the women. If she was pregnant and delivered a child, and from the paternity tests if the child is likely to be hers. Such evidence is useful only in those cases where the age of the suppositious child does not correspond to the date of the pretended pregnancy and subsequent delivery.[1-4]

In 1922 a case occurred at Ahmedabad, where a young widow abducted with the help of a nurse, from the Victoria Jubilee Hospital, a newly born child who she passed off as her own alleging that it had been born after her husband's death (posthumous child and pretended delivery while in fact she had had none. In October 1923, a Bhatia widow[3] of Bombay was sentenced to one year's simple imprisonment and a fine of Rs,2000 for having tried with the help of two accomplices, to conceal the fact of her giving birth of female twins soon after her husband's death by substituting male child and claiming a share in the property of her husband. The two accomplices were also sentenced to various terms of imprisonment.[4]

INFANTICIDE (INFANT DEATHS)
According to the infanticide Act of England (1938), **infanticide** means the unlawful killing of a child under the age of one year. Only the mother can be charged with the offence, when the circumstances justify it, such as when the infant is killed by its mother while suffering from disease of the mind due the effect of stress associated with her pregnancy, delivery, puerperium or location. In such cases the mother may not be held wholly responsible for killing the infant. In India there is no such special Act, and as such there is no distinction between the murder of newborn infant and that of any other individual. **Foeticide** is the killing of the foetus at any time prior to birth. **Neonaticide** is the deliberate killing of a child within 4 week of its birth. **Filicide** is the killing of a child by its parents. Infanticide does not include the death of foetus during labour, when it is destroyed by craniotomy or decapitation. Infanticide is the rare, and usually committed by a young unmarried woman or widow. Infanticide is usually committed at the time of, or within in a few minutes or hours after the birth. The alleged mother should be examined for signs of recent delivery.

STILLBIRTH: A stillborn child is one which is born after 28 weeks of pregnancy, and which did not breathe or show any other signs of life, at any time after being completely born. The child was alive in uterus, but dies during the process of birth. Stillbirths occur more frequently among illegitimate, immature male children in primiparae. The incident is about five percent. It is born in sterile condition, and as such, putrefaction to starts on the surface and extends inward, where in case of newly born child which lived for some time, the bacteria inside the body may cause putrefaction to start in the abdomen. Signs of prolonged labour, i.e. oedema and bleeding into the scalp, and severe moulding of the head indicate stillbirth or death from natural causes shortly after birth.[6]

DEADBIRTH: A deadborn child is one which had died in utero and shows one of the following signs after it is completely born.

> **(1) Rigor mortis at delivery.**
>
> **(2) Maceration:** Maceration **is** a process of aseptic autolysis, and is the usual change. This occurs when dead child remains in the uterus for about three to four days surrounded with liquor amnii but the exclusion of air. Signs of maceration are not seen if the child is born within 24 hours after death. If air enters the liquior amnii after death of the foetus, putrefaction occurs instead of maceration.
>
> The ealiest sign of maceration is skin slippage, which can be seen in 12 hours after the death of the child in utero. Gas in aorta (in 12 hours) of foetus indicates foetal death. Collapse of the vertebral column occur. The body of a macerated foetus is soft, flaccid and flattens out when placed on a level surface. It has a sweetish, disagreeable odour. The skin is red or purple. Large blebs appear at 24 hours, which contain a red serous or serosanguineous fluid. The epidermis detaches easily and leaves moist and greasy areas. The tissues are oedematous. The abdomen is distended. The serous cavaties may contain a turbid reddish fluid. The bones are flexible and readily detached from soft parts. The joins become abnormally mobile. The skull bones are separated and oedematous and lose their morphology, but lungs and uterus remain unchanged for a long time. The umbilical cord is red, smooth thickened and soft.
>
> **Spalding's Sign :** Loss of alignment and overriding of the bones of the cranial vault occurs due to shrinkage of the cerebrum after death of the foetus. In the early stage, there is only loss of alignment without overriding .The sign will develop earlier with a vertex presentation than with a breech. It may be detеched within a few days of death of the foetus, but often takes much longer time sometimes two to three weeks.
>
> **(3) Mummification:** Mummification occurs when foetus dies from defiant supply of blood, when liquor amnii is scanty, and when no air enters uterus.

VIABILITY OF THE INFANT: Viability means the physical ability of a foetus to lead a separate existence after birth apart from its mother, by virtue of a certain degree of development. A child is viable after 210 days of intrauterine life, and in some cases after 180.

LIVEBIRTH: It means that the child showed signs of the life when only part of the child was out of mother, though the child may not have breathed or completely born. The causing of death of such a child is regarded as murder.

SIGNS OF LIVEBIRTH

In civil cases, any sign of life after complete birth of the child is accepted as proof of livebirth e.g., hearing a cry, seeing movement of the body or limbs, muscle contraction, etc. A child may cry either in the uterus or in the vagina which may be heard by bystanders or even outside the room of delivery. This occurs only when the membranes have ruptured and air has entered the uterus. The law presumes that every newborn child found dead was born dead until the contrary is proved. In criminal cases, signs of livebirth have to be demonstrated by post-mortem examination of the child.

Shape of the Chest : Before respiration ,the chest is flat and its circumference is one to two cm. less than the abdomen at the level of the umbilicus. After respiration, the chest expands and become arched or drum-shaped.

The Position of the Diaphragm: The abdomen should be opened before the thorax, and the highest point of the diaphragm is noted , which is found about the level of fourth or fifth rib if respiration has not taken , and at the level of the sixth or seventh rib after breathing. The Position is affected by gases of decomposition.

Lungs: Breathing causes important and permanent changes in the lungs. The extent of which depends on the physical strength and period of respiration.

   (1) **Volume:** Unrespired lungs appear smaller, being collapsed on to the hilum when the thorax is opened. Fully respired lungs fill the pleural cavities, and the medical edges overlap the mediastinum and part of the pericardium.
   (2) **Margins:** Before respiration the margins are sharp, which become rounded even when breathing is feeble. Glistening bullae appear along the margin when there has been a struggle to breathe due to some mechanical obstruction.
   (3) **Consistency:** Before respiration the lungs are dens, firm and non-crepitant like liver. After respiration they are soft, elastic ,spongy and

crepitant. The lungs are also crepitant in putrefaction and after artificial inflation.

(4) **Color and Expansion of the Air-sacs: B**efore respiration they are uniform reddish-brown or bluish-red, according to the degree of anoxia.The surface of the lobules is marked with shallow furrows. On section, interior of the lungs is uniform in color and texture, and little frothless blood exudes on pressure. After respiration, the air cells become distended with air. As the air vesicles expand, they become raised slightly above the surface, and may be seen as polygonal or angular areas on the surface of the lungs, giving it a fine mosaic appearance. As the blood becomes aerated in the expanded . area the color become a light red or pink, and the whole lung has a mottled or marbled appearance with rose –colored patches of expansion and aeration alternation with the collapsed dark bluish-red area. On section, frothy blood exudes from the cut surface on slight pressure. Bloodstained froth in bronchi and bronchioles indicates that respiration has taken place.

(5) **Blood in the Lungs Beds:** The amount of blood in the lungs after respiration is about twice that in circulation before respiration.

(6) **Weight: (A) Statics Test or Fodere's Test:** The lungs are ligated their hila and separated. The average weight of both lungs before respiration varies from 30 to 40 g. and after respiration from 60 to 66 g . The increase in weight is due to the increased flow of blood.

(B) **Ploucquet's test:** The blood flow in the long beds is so increased after breathing that their weight is almost doubled, from 1/70 of the body weight before respiration to 1/35 after respiration. The increment in weight is not constant and is not a reliable indicator of breathing.

(7) **The Hydrostatic Test:** It is based on the fact that on breathing, the volume of the lungs is increased which of the body additional body, due to which their specific gravity is diminished. The specific gravity of the lungs before respiration varies from 1040 to 1050 and after respiration about 940. A ligaute is tied on the bronchi, and lungs separated .Each lung individually is placed in water. If they float each lung is cut into 12 to 20 pieces and placed in water. If these pieces, float they are each squeezed in between thumb and index finger under the surface of water, to see if any bubbles of air escape and if they still persist to float; or they are taken out of water wrapped in a piece of cloth and air. The pieces are again placed in water and if they continue to float due the presence of residual air it indicate that respiration has taken place. If the pieces sink after pressure respiration has not taken place. If some pieces float while other sinks, it shows feeble respiration.[1,6]

The expanded lungs may sink from: (1) Disease, e.g. acute oedema, pneumonia, conggential syphilis, etc. (2) **Atelectasis** (non-expansion) of the lungs due to: (1) Air is not entering the lungs due to feeble respiration but aeration of lungs may occur through the mucosa of trachea and bronchi. (2) Complete absorption of air from the lungs by the blood, it circulation continued after stoppage of respiration than what is inhaled during inspiration. (4) Obstruction by an alveolar duct membrane.

The unexpanded lungs may float from :(1) Putrefactive gases. (2) Artificial inflation: The foetal lungs may be artificial inflated by blowing air through a tube, catheter or cannula passed into the trachea or by the mouth-to-mouth method. In such case, the lungs can be inflated only partially and the stomach contains air.

Hydrostatic test is not necessary when: (1) The foetus is a monster. (2) The foetus is macerated or mummified. (3) The foetus is born before 180days of gestation. (4) The stomach contains milk (5) The umbilical cord has separated and a scar formed.

Respiration Before and during Birth:

A child may breath (1) while it is in the uterus, after the rupture of the membranes **(vatigus uterinus)** (2) while its head is in the vagina **(vagitus vaginalis),** (3) while its head is protruding from the outlet. A child which has breathed in the uterus or vagina may die from natural causes, before it is completely born. Therefore, **proof of breathing is not proof of livebirth**. In the new born child, the respiration may not be strong or deep enough to expand the air cells and the child may live for some time on oxygen absorbed from the respiratory cells of the alveolar ducts. Some air may pass into cells, may not be sufficient to distend the fibrous tissue. This air may be absorbed by the blood, or may be lost. The child may live for many hours or even one or two days with only small portion of its lung tissue expanded. When the air cell have been distended once they never return foetal condition. For the above reasons the hydrostatic test fails in a small percentage of cases.

Microscopic Examination of the lungs:

Microscopic examination is of value in determining the extent of respiration and the presence of pulmonary disease or abnormality, which may have caused or contributed to the death. At full term, the normal foetal lung is almost completely atelectic, but may of its terminal bronchioles and vesicles are partly expanded by amniotic fluid. The material is not stained with haemotoxlin and eosin giving the impression that alveoli have been well expanded by air. In a child who has breathed, diffuse atelectasis may be seen. It was thought that if respiration has not taken place, the alveoli appear as hollow gland-like structures lined by cuboidal or columnar epithelium, but if respiration has taken place, the alveoli are well expended and lined by flattened epithelium. This is not correct for the change in the type of cell which lines the air sacs does not occur with the onset of respiration. If the child has lived only for a few minutes microscopy cannot always provide clear evidence of extra-utrerine respiration obstruction of the lower bronchial tree by hyaline duct membrane causes respiration failure. The struggle to breathe may result in (1) incomplete lung expansion, (2) suboxia and cyanosis; (3) petechial haemorrhages mainly subpleural, (4) oedema of the mediastinum and often of the lung.

(IV) Changes in the Stomach and Intestine:

Air is swallowed into the stomach during respiration. The stomach and intestines are removed after trying double ligature at each end. They float in water if respiration has taken place, otherwise they sink. This is known as **Breslau's second life or stomach-bowel test**. This test is not of much value, because air may be swallowed by the child in attempting to free the air-passage of fluid obstructions in cases of stillbirth. It is useless when there in decomposition. When dissected under water the stomach shows mucus, saliva and air bubbles if respiration has taken place and only mucus if breathing has not occurred. Blood, meconium or liquor amnii in the stomach indicate that the child was alive at or shortly before birth. If milk is presence in the stomach it is positive evidence that the child has lived for some time after birth.

(V) Changes in the Middle Ear (Wredin's Test):

Before Birth the middle ear contains gelatinous embryonic connective tissue. With respiration the sphincter at the pharyngeal end of Eustachian tubes relaxes and air replaces the gelatinous substance in few hours to five weeks. This is not all reliable.

Livebirth is brobable when:

1. All the lobes of the lungs are fully expanded.
2. There is oedema of the lungs, specially gross.
3. An alveolar duct membrane is present and has widespread distribution in the lungs.
4. Pulmonary atelectasis due to obstration by the alveolar duct membrane is present.

5. Contusions of the lungs are present.

Stillbirth is probablein the presence of:
(1) Maceration of the infant.
(2) Flooding of the lungs with liquor amnii, and specially evidence of phagocytosis of meconium by the cells lining the air sacs.
(3) Desquamation of bronichial epithelium.
(4) Distention of large bowel with meconium indicating a struggle to breathe.

(VI) Other Signs: Several changes occur in the child after, which are helpful in estimating the length of time the child lived after birth.

(1) **Blood:** Nucleated red cells usally disappear from the blood within 24 hours. Foetal haemoglobin (synthesized mainly in the liver) which is about 80 to 90 percent before birth rapidly decreases to 7 to 8 percent at third month.

(2) **Meconium: It** is the green sticky substance consisting of thickened bile and mucus. The meconium is completely excreted from the large intestine in the first 24 to 48 hours after birth, but in breech presentation and also in severe anoxia, the meconium may be excreted completely before birth. Meconium stains are brownish-green and stiffen the cloth. The reaction is acid.

(3) **Caput Succedaneum: This** is an area of soft swelling that forms in the scalp over the presenting part of the head in vertex presentation. The elevated, rounded area of the caput succedaneum corresponding to the portion of the scalp surface that is exposed within the opening of the dilated cervix during labour. The scalp in the area of the caput is swollen to three to four times it is normal thickness due to oedema and congestion, due to local interface with venous return produced by the pressure of the rigid cervical ring. Most commonly the caput succedaneum gradually diminished within a weak often disappearing during the first day after birth.

Cephalhaematoma: This is a localized accumulation of blood deep to the scalp, between the periosteum and bone surface. The haematoma is limited to the periosteal sheath of a single bone commonly the right parietal bone and never crosses a suture line. Cephalhaematoma is rare occurring in less than one percent of newborns, and varies in size from one to 5 cm. The haematoma swelling often tends to increase during the first day or two after birth as more and more blood accumulates, but gradually shrinks in subsequent week as the blood is absorbed.

(4) **Skin:** At first the skin is bright-red which becomes darker on second or third day, then brick-red yellow and normal in about a week. **Vernix caseosa** covers the skin mostly in the axilla, inguinal region and folds of the neck buttocks and persists for one or two days. Sometimes it may be absent at birth and it removed by washing. The skin of the abdomen shed in flakes during the first three days after birth.

(5) **Umbilical Cord:** The blood clots in the cut end two hours after birth and the vessels begin to be closed in about 24 hours. The cord attached to the child shrinks and dries in 12 to 24 hours (but this appearance is also seen in the body of a stillborn oinfant) and an inflammatory ring forms at its base in 36 to 48 hours. It contacts and mummifies on second or third day. Mummification of the cord also occurs after death if exposed to air. The cord falls off on the fifth or sixth day leaves an uncer which heals and forms a scar in 10 to 12 days.

(6) **Circulation:** Contraction of the umbilical arteries starts in about ten hours and is completely closed by third day. The umbilical vein and ductus venosus are closed on the fourth day. The ductus arteriosus closed by tenth day and foramen ovale by second or third month.

CAUSES OF DEATH:
Natural Causes:

(1) Immaturity. (2) Debility due to lack of general development. (3) Congenital diseases e.g, syphilis and disease of the child's internal organs, such as lungs, heart, Brain, etc (4) Malformations. (5) Haemorrhage from the umbilical cord genital organs, stomach, rectum etc. (6) Post-maturity. (7) Pre-eclamptic toxaemia. (8) Disease of the placenta or its accidental separation from the uterine wall. (9) Placenta praeyia or abnormal gestation. (10) Neonatal infection. (11) Intrapartum or ante-partum anoxia. (12) Cerebral birth trauma. (13)Erythroblastosis

UNNATURAL CAUSES: These are may be:

 (I)Accidental, and (II) Criminal.

Accidental Causes: (A) During Birth:**(1) Prolonged labour:** Severe compression of the head against contracted or deformed pelvis may cause intracranial haemorrhage and death with or without fissured fracture of the parietal bones. Subdural haemorrhages are common and usually bilateral. Tentorial tears may be bilateral and haemorrhage occur into the subdural space

265

either above or below the tentorium. In such cases the head of the child shows evidence of well-developed moulding and caput succedaneum. Fracture and dislocations of the limb bones and clavicles may be found.

(2) Prolapse of the cord or pressure on the cord produces death by asphysia. The cord is liable to be compressed by the foetal head, specially in breech presentations.

(3) Twisting of the cord round the neck or knots of the cord causes strangulation.

(4) Injuries to the Mother: Heavy blows or Knicks or the mother' abdomen or falls from a height may cause concussion of the brain of the child, with or without fracture of skull or rupture of blood vessels or organs. Rarely powerful uterine constructions may fracture the cranial bones of the foetus

Death of the Mother: The child can be saved, if it can be delivered within five to ten minutes of the mother death.

After Birth: (1) Suffocation: It may result when the membranes cover the head during birth or if the face is pressed accidentally in the cloth or submerged in the discharges, such as blood liquor amnii or meconium. Achild can survive in the membranes for 20 to 30 minutes.

Precipitate Labour: Labour terminating in a very short time than that taken on the average, either by primipara or multipara is called precipitate labour. In this delivery occurs suddenly and rapidly without the knowledge of the mother. All the three stages of labour are merged into one. The foetus is normal or premature. It is possible in multipara with large roomy pelves, but is extremely rare in primipara. Sometimes a women may not be   able to distinguish the sence of fullness produced by the descend of a child, from the feeling of bulky evacuation. The child may die from (1) suffocation by falling into a lavatory pan, (2) head injury and fracture of the skull with subdural haemorrhage often bilateral by a fall on a hard floor, if the woman was standing and (3) haemorrhage from the torn end of the cord.

If the birth occur into the toilet bowl, or into a bucket containing liquid , the infant will inhale the liquid and blood and meconium and viginal macus are found in the air passages. In accidental falls the haemorrhage are usually subdural and often bilateral. The average length of a cord is 50 cm which is not sufficient to allow the child to fall to the ground and is sufficiently strong to withstand the weight of the foetus without breaking. The cord is torn most commonly at the foetal end than the placentral end, But is not torn in its middle. The torn edges are ragged. Caput succedaneum and moulding of the head are absent. Foreign material such as mud, sand, gravel, may be found in the hair or injured scalp of the child. The fractures of the skull are usually fissured and limited to parietal bones but may extend to frontal and squamous part of temporal bones.

Medico-legal Importance: (1) The mother or her relative may be accused of killing the infant while the death may be due to injury, haemorrhage or asphyxia from precipitate labour. (2) In a case of infant murder, death may be attributed to participated labour.

(2) Criminal Causes: (A) Acts of Commission: They are act done positively to causes the death of the infant.

(1) Suffocation: This is commonly caused by pressing the face into a pillow or by a hand. Overlaying, or forcing mud rag or cotton-wool into the mouth are other method.

(2) Strangulation: Throttling or strangulation by a ligature is also common and in the latter case the ligature is frequently left in situ. Sometimes umbilical cord is used as a ligature to simulate accident.

(3) Drowning: It is rare but the body of a dead foetus may be thrown into a well tank, etc.

(4) Burning: Burning is rare but it may be used is a mode of disposal.

(5) Blunt Head Injury: Dashing the head against a well or the floor by holding the feet is rare. Blows on head may be produced with a blunt weapon. Subdural and subarachnoid by fractures (depressed or comminuted) of the skull and contusions and laceration of the brain and scalp.

(6) Fractures and dislocation of cervical vertebrae: These may be caused by twisting the neck.

(7) Wounds: The child may be killed by stabs, incised wounds, cut-throat, etc.

(8) Poisoning: Rare.

Acts of Omission or Neglect: A woman is guilty of criminal negligence, if she does not take ordinary precaution to save her child after birth. The following acts of omission amount to crime. (1) Failure to provide proper assistance during labour may causes death by suffocation or head injury. (2) Failure to tie the cord after it is cut may cause death by haemorrhage. (3) Failure to clear the air passages which may be obstructed by amniotic fluid or mucus. Failure to protect the child from exposure to heat or cold. (5)Failure to supply the child with proper food.

BATTERED BABY SYNDROME OR NON-ACCIDENTAL INJURY OF CHILDHOOD:

It is also known as child abuse syndrome, Caffey's syndrome and maltreatment syndrome in children. The typical form of this condition is very rare in India. A battered child is one who has received repetitive physical injuries as a result of non-accidental violence produced by a parent or guardian. In additional to physical injury there may be non-accidental deprivation of nutrition care and affection. The classical features of syndrome are obvious disagreement between the nature of the injuries and explanation offered by the parents and delay between the injury and medical attention which cannot be explained. This constant feature is repetitive of injuries at different dates often progressing from minor to more serve.

Features: (1) Age: Usually less than three years **(2) Sex:** Slightly more in male (55 to 63%)

Position in Family: One child of a family commonly the eldest or the youngest and often unwanted, such as the result of pregnancy before marriage, failure of contraception or illegitimate child **(4) Socio-economic factors:** Parents tend to be young between 20 to 30 year, and belong to lower social class and lower education. The family is usually isolated. There is often a history of family disharmony, long-standing emotional problems, or financial problems. Many mothers have multiple social and psychiatric problems. The mother is of lower I.Q., often pregnant or in the premenstrual period at the time of battering. Most of the parents suffer guilt-amnesia. **(5) History:** The is obvious difference between the nature of the injuries and the explanation offered by the parents, which may change on several times of repetition, each time the child is taken to a different doctor. **(6) Treatment**: There is always unexplainable delay between the injury and medical attention.

Injuries: Soft tissue injuries are very common. Laceration of the mucosa inside the upper lip, often tear of fraenulum, is the most characteristic lesion. Multiple bruies of various ages all over the body from rough handling, or beating, kicking or throwing the infant are common. Caffey (1974) described the effects of shaking a child as a major cause of subdural haematoma and intraocular bleeding in battered babies the so-called **"infantile whiplash syndrome".** Recent research has thrown doubt on the common acceptance of this mechanism. In such cases, bruies are produced in areas where the child is held by the hands but there are no external injuries to the head or fractures. Permanent brain damage may be caused due to habitual prolonged shacking. Bites marks may be found on the cheeks, shoulders, chest abdomen arms, legs and buttocks. Bruies are usually present around the elbows and knees due to gripping of the child so as to shake or pull him, or hurl him into cot or against furniture, etc, Subgaleal haematoma resulting from vigorous pulling on the scalp is characteristic. **Visceral injuries:** Subdural haematoma is found in about 40% of fatal cases. Crushing or compressing forces applied to the abdomen produce either "brusting" injuries of the lever or spleen or perforation of distended hollow viscera including the stomach, intestine or urinary bladder. Small circular pitted burn may indicate deliberate stubbing of cigarette ends upon the skin. The violence force applied to the limbs involve pulling and twisting, both capable of producing epiphyseal sepration and periosteal shearing. Long bone fracture result from compression, bending and direct forcible blows. Anteroposterior compression of the chest causes fracture of ribs midaxillary line. Violent squeezing of the chest from side to side causes fracture at the costochondral junctions. Multiple rib fracture also occurs along the posterior angles of the ribs. After about two weeks callus is formed and on X-ray a "string of beads" appearance is seen in the paravertebral gutting (**nobbing fractures).** Before autopsy a whole body X-ray should be taken to detect old fractures.

Diagnosis: The diagnosis depends upon (1) nature of injuries, (2) time taken to seek medical advice, and (3) recurrent injuries. Differential diagnosis has to be made from scurvy, congential syphilis, infantile cortical hyperostosis and osteogenesis imperfect.

MUNCHAUSEN'S SYNDROME BY PROXY: Munchausen syndrome is feigning illness or injury and going from hospital to hospital for unnecessary investigation and treatment. These patients appear to be compulsively driven to make their complaints. The person is aware that he is acting an illness. But he cannot stop act.

Munchausen's syndrome by proxy is a variant which is very peculiar and dangerous type of child abuse usually involving the mother, in which and symptoms of illness with a fictious history. The child is admitted frequently in the hospital for medical evaluation for the non-existent conditions.

Method of simulation or production of illness: (1) The mother pricks her finger and adds blood to the urine of the child and takes the sample to the doctor. (2) The mother gives insulin to the child takes to hospital with hypoglycaemia. (3) The child's nose is closed with two fingers and the lower jaw pushed up with the palm to block the airway. (4) A pillow or towel is put over the face of the child and the face is pushed down into bed clothing. (5) Vomiting: allegation or by ipecacuanha. (6) Diarrhoea: laxatives or salt poisoning. (7) CNS depression: barbiturates, benzodiazipines. (8) Fever alleged (9) Rash: scratching or intoxication.

SUDDEN INFANT DEATH SYNDROME: Sudden infant death syndrome (SIDS), or cot death or crib death is defined as the sudden and unexpected death of a healthy infant whose death remains unexplained even after a complete autopsy.

Feature: (1) Incidence: 0.6 per 1000 livebirths. (2) **Ages:** Two week to two years Majority of cases occur between one and 7 months with a marked peak between two to three months (3) **Sex:** There is slight increase in the males. (4) **Twins:** There is increased risk (threefold) amongst members of twin pair. Most twins are premature and of low birth weight. (5) **Geographical distribution:** The occurrence is worldwide. (6) **Times of Death:** Death always occurs during sleep at all times of night with a moderate increase in the early morning hours. (7) **Social-economic standard** of the family is usually low.

The child is either quite well when put to the bed or may have only a minor upper respiratory tract infection (cold and snuffles) or minor gastrointestinal disturbances. Cold death are major causes of death in infants in the first six months of life.

Autopsy: Milk or a bloodstained fronth is sometimes seen on the child's mouth, nostrils, or bedding. The post-modern finding are completely negative. In about 15% of cases some pathological condition may be found such as frank pneumonia congenital heart disease, Down's syndrome or a tracheobronchitis. The only constant findings are multiple petechial haemorrhages on the visceral surface of the heart lugs and thymus which are agonal in nature perhaps from terminal respiratory effort against closed glottis. Peribronichial cell infiltraction is the main finding. A small amount of milk vomit in the trachea and main bronchi and shedding of individual tracheobronchial epithelial cells are commonly found. Many infants show froth in the air-passages and facial pallor.

The lungs show patchy or uniform purplish discolouration of the surface and are firm in consistency with congestion, oedema and increase in weight.

Theories: There is no single cause for cot death and many deaths may result from a number of causes. Some infant have prolonged **"sleep apnoea"** (a periodic failure to breathe during sleep), which makes them susceptible to hypoxia, which leads to bradycardia and cardiac arrest. But this has not been substantiated. Respiratory infection may produce a viraemia, which adds to the sleep depression of the respiratory centres. Nasal oedema and mucus secretion may further narrow the small upper respiratory passages and in some hypotonic babies, a flaccid pharynx and even neck posture may further reduce the airway. Staphylococcus aureus infection of upper respiratory tract is said to cause anaphylactic shock and sudden death. An element of laryngeal spasm has also been suggested. Whatever the cause, factor is pregnancy that inhibit foetal circulation could damage the child's brain, so that it is no longer control breathing properly. An unidentified trigger could affect the airway of a sleeping infant. The brain would not respond correctly and breathing would stop. There is no single cause of cot death, and death may result from a number of causes which combine and act via a common pathway of cardiorespiratory failure.

Other causes of death which have been proposed are: conduction system anomalies, defective or immature respiratory or cardiac control centres, adrenal insufficiency, hypersensitivity to cow's milk parathyroid deficiency, selenium deficiency, vitamin E deficiency, antibody deficiency, hypogammaglobulinaemia, metabolic disorders, anaphylactic shock, etc.

REFERENCE
1. Parikh, C.K., Parikh's textbook of medical jurisprudence forensic medicine and toxicology, sixth edition (2011), C.B.S. Publishers and Distributors, 4596/1A, Darya Ganj, New Delhi-110002 (India).
2. Gupta A.K., Essentials of Forensic Medicine and Toxicology, Fifth edition, Current Books International, 60, Lenin Saranee, Kolkata-700013.
3. Mahanta Pautul, Modern Textbook of Forensic Medicine & Toxicology (2014), Jaypee Brothers Medical Publishers (P) Ltd., New Delhi.
4. Modi, N.J. Medical Jurisprudence and Toxicology, Twentieth Edition (1977), N.M. Tripathi Private Limited, Bombay.
5. Biswas Gautam, Review of Forensic Medicine & Toxicology, Second Edition (2012), Jaypee Brothers Medical Publishers (P) Ltd., New Delhi.
6. Krishan Vij Textbook of Forensic medicine and Toxicology, 4th Edt.

Chapter 23

SEXUAL OFFENCES

SEXUAL OFFENCES

Sexual offences

Sexual offences are acts of illegal sexual intercourse with another person or with an animal or any other illegal act to obtain sexual gratification.

Classification:

1. Natural offences: It includes Sex-linked offences Indecent :-(a) those offences which are assault: - Any offence committed on committed in order of a female with the intension or nature, i.e. penetration of knowledge to outrage her modesty vagina by the penis (b) Sexual perversions: - Sexual perversions Rape, Incest & Adultery are habitual acts to obtain sexual

2. Unnatural offences: Unnatural sexual offences include;

1 -Sodomy
2- Tribadism/ lesbianism
3- Bestiality
4- Buccal/oral coitus

These offences are punishable under SEC 377 I.P.C.with an imprisonment for life or with imprisonment which may extend to 10 years or fine. Furthermore, the offences are cognizable, non bailiable, non- compoundable and tried by magistrate of first class. In a trial of an accused under this section, the prosecution must prove that the:
i- Accused had carnal intercourse with a man, woman or an animal.
ii- Such intercourse was against the order of nature.
iii- The act was done voluntarily by the accused.
iv-Pentration had occurred.

RAPE

IPC 375Rape is defined as unlawful sexual intercourse by a man with his wife under the age of 15 years, with any woman under the age of 16years, or above that age, against her will, without her consent, or with her consent when it has been obtained by unlawful means.

RAPE: IPC 375 With his wife under the age of 15 years

RAPE: IPC 375 Any other women under the age of 16 years with/without her consent

RAPE: IPC 375 Any other women above the age of 16 years against her will, without her consent(3a) when her consent has been obtained by putting her or any person in whom she is interested in fear of death or of hurt.

RAPE: IPC 375 With her consent (3b) when the man knows that he is not her husband, and that her consent is given because she believes that he is another man to whom she is or believes herself to be lawfully married.

RAPE: IPC 375 With her consent(3c), when, at the time of giving such consent, by reason of unsoundness of mind or intoxication or the administration by him personally or through another of any stupefying or unwholesome substance, she is unable to understand the nature and consequences of that to which she consents.

RAPE: IPC 375 Exception If the wife is above 15 years of age, sex without her consent and will, is not rape, Sexual intercourse by a man with his wife, the wife not being under 15 years of age, is not rape.

Constitutes Rape• Male private parts inserted into female, no rule extent of depth• Need not be completed act of intercourse• Slightest penetration of penis within vulva, with or without emission of semen or rupture of hymen.• Committed even when inability to produce penile erection.• No age limit for accused – potency decided by court based on evidence.

376 IPC: Punishment for Rape: Punishment for rape may extend from seven years to life imprisonment along with fine. If the woman raped is his wife and is not under 12 years, the imprisonment may extend to 2 years with/without fine.

376 IPC: Punishment for Rape: When the victim not being the wife, is below 16yrs, sexual intercourse amounts to rape and is called; Statutory Rape. (Question of consent or non-consent does not arise)

376A IPC: Punishment for Rape: Intercourse by a man with his wife during separation shall be punished with imprisonment of either description for a term which may extend to two years and shall also be liable to fine.

376B IPC: Punishment for Rape: Intercourse by public servant with woman in his custody :-(custodial rape) -shall be punished with imprisonment of either description for a term which may extend to five years and shall also be liable to fine.

376C IPC: Punishment for Rape: Intercourse by superintendent of jail, remand home, etc. shall be punished with imprisonment of either description for a term which may extend to five years and shall also be liable to fine.

376D IPC: Punishment for Rape: Intercourse by any member of the management or staff of a hospital with any woman in that hospital:- shall be punished with imprisonment of either description for a term which may extend to five years and shall also be liable to fine.

Gang Rape: Where a woman is raped by one or more in a group of persons shall be punished with rigorous imprisonment for a term which shall not be less than ten years but which may be for life and shall also be liable to fine.

PROCEDURE FOR EXAMINATION OF VICTIM

Informed Consent: Informed consent of the victim should be taken in writing in presence of a witness if she above the age of 12 years. (In India) if she is under the age of 12 years or a mentally subnormal person, the written consent of the parents or guardian should be taken. SECTION 90 IPC Consent of insane person.-if the consent is given by a person who, from unsoundness of mind, or intoxication, is unable to understand the nature and consequence of that to which he gives his consent; or Consent of child unless the contrary appears from the context, if the consent is given by a person who is under twelve years of age. The examination should be made in the presence of a female nurse or a female relation unless the doctor is female. (Section 53(2) OF CrPC) whenever a female is to be examined, the examination should be made only by, or under the supervision of, a female registered medical practitioner.

The principal features of the examination are: Preliminary data, The statement of the victim and others separately, Signs of struggle on clothes and body, Examination of the genitals for Local signs of violation, Genital injuries,

Presence of spermatozoa and other microorganisms, Any evidence of STD , Collection of laboratory specimens , Inference , and advice on follow-up.

Preliminary data: This includes name in full, address, age, occupation and social status, date, time of arrival, consent for examination, identification marks, by whom examination is requested, and the name of the female nurse present at the time of examination.

The statement: The statement of the victim in her words must be written down as much as possible "Word for Word". The amount of violence used, the position of the assailant, and the mode of attack should be elicited. It is necessary to inquire if vaginal, oral, or rectal contact occurred. Her statement should be noted with reference to Pain, Haemorrhage, Sensation as to penetration and emission and the appearance of discharge If she cried for help, or was too terrified to do so, or she fainted Enquiry should be made of the events after the alleged assault, e. g, if she has changed her clothing, bathed or passed urine. Any delay in making complain to the authorities should have a proper explanation. A record should be made of the statement of others who accompany her. The degree of agreement of the various statements is important.

Signs of struggle on clothes and body: These should be looked for on the clothes and the body. The clothing, if are the same as that worn at the time of crime should be examined in good light for evidence of a struggle, such as tears in the fabrics, marks of mud or grass, or stain of blood or semen. When clothes are torn, corresponding injuries to the body may be present and should be looked for. Mud and blood stains, when present, are generally seen on the back clothes while seminal stains are seen on the front clothes. Stains may be found on the material, e.g. Handkerchief, used for cleaning after the assault. When blood stains are seen, it must be ascertained if they are due to menstruation.

On microscopic examination, menstrual blood is found to contain endometrial cells from the uterus, epithelial cells from the vagina, and a large number of microorganisms which are not found in ordinary blood. Trichomonas vaginalis or monilia may be present. Blood should be taken for grouping and DNA characteristics to determine if the stains belong to the victim or assailant. Seminal stains should also be grouped to ascertain subsequently if they match with the assailant's blood group. The clothing should be retained, carefully dried, labelled, and forwarded to the Forensic Science Laboratory for examination of suspicious stains, either blood, semen, or both.

Examination of the genitals for Local signs of violation and genital injuries:
The presence or absence of blood stains about the legs or vagina should be observed and if present, should be ascertained whether such stains could be due to menstruation, or blood from the victim or assailant. If dry, they should be scraped with a clean blunt scalpel and preserved for examination. The pubic hair should be examined for matting from seminal fluid or blood, and for foreign hairs. If the hairs are matted together, a portion must be cut off and kept for examination. The pubic hair should be combed out to collect non-matching male pubic hair and a comparison sample of plucked hair preserved for laboratory examination. Some believe that hair need not be plucked and that cutting would be alright provided all other foreign hairs have been removed by combing, etc.

Examination of genitals should take in good light and, when possible, in lithotomy position, with the parts fully exposed. The sooner the examination is made the better, and menstruation should not be a cause for delay. The vulva, hymen, vagina and the perineum should be examined for any injuries. To determine the degree of hymenal rupturing and whether this is recent or old, a glass rod with a small spherical head (Glaister Knee Rod), warmed to body temperature, if possible transilluminated, may be introduced into the vagina and partial withdrawn to display the edge of hymen. Signs of recent rupture are ragged tears in the hymen with lack of epithelial healing, but with oedema and haemorrhage. Women who pay no attention to the cleanliness of their genital region often have superficial areas of erythema, irritation and occasionally abrasions, and therefore any superficial injuries found in this area must be carefully assessed in the light of personal hygiene of the woman. Redness due to long standing inflammation or to irritation by a chronic discharge must be distinguished from the effect of recent injury. It must be noted at this stage, if gait is normal. When genital injury is present, the gait is broad based and painful.

The dispensability of the vagina should be noted in relation to the number of fingers it can admit without causing discomfort. If it can admit two fingers easily, sexual intercourse has probably occurred. The extent of violence to the private parts will depend upon the age of the victim and her previous condition with reference to intercourse, whether virgin, sexually active, or a child. Slaughter states that colposcopic examination, within 72 hours of assault, is an important adjunct to traditional simple macroscopic assessment of genital trauma.

RAPE ON A VIRGIN

Rape on a virgin: Any bruising, laceration or swelling of the vulva is noted. The labia are then opened by gentle traction in order to examine the hymen for rupture. Laceration of this structure occurs with the first intercourse, and in a virgin this is the principal evidence of the crime. The character and extent of the injury will vary in different cases depending upon the nature of the hymen, disproportion between male and female parts, extent of penetration, and amount of force used. With the first intercourse, tearing of hymen usually occurs posteriorly at one or other side or in the middle. The semi lunar often ruptures on both sides. The annular hymen which closes up the vaginal which nearly closes up the vaginal orifice may suffer several tears. The fourchette is torn and the fossa navicularis disappears. Even the posterior commissure may be ruptured. The latter injury usually does not occur in consenting sexual intercourse unless there is much disproportion between the male and female parts.

Soon after the act, the torn margins are sharp and red, and bleed on touch. Even when examined after 3 to 4 days of offence, the edges of laceration are congested and swollen. The surrounding tissues are tissues are also swollen and tender. With violent intercourse, laceration of vaginal wall invariably occurs posteriorly or slightly posteriorly. The gait is broad based and painful. In indecent assault, due to digital penetration, the laceration is usually single, may be lateral, and is often incomplete.

Presence of Spermatozoa and other Microorganisms: Normally, sperms remain motile in the vagina for about 6-8 hours and occasionally for 12 hours. Non-motile forms are detectable for about 24 hours with occasional reports to 48-72 and very rarely 96 hours. Motility persists longer at body temperature. The sperms remain motile in the uterus cavity for 3-5 days. Non-motile sperms remain in the uterine cavity for weeks or months after death. To demonstrate the presence of sperms, the vaginal contents are aspirated by means of a blunt-ended pipette. A wet preparation is then made on a slide and examined under a microscope for motile spermatozoa. If motile sperms are seen, it would mean that intercourse has taken place within about 12 hours. If the sperms are not motile, it is not possible to say exactly when intercourse took place except that it may be over 12 hours and within 24-48 hours and occasionally up to 72 hours. Intact sperms are rarely found in the vagina after 72 hours of coitus. In such a case, sperms heads and tails can be separately demonstrated by using picroindigocarmine which stain sperms heads "Red" and tails "Green and Red". A smear is also made from the vaginal contents, fixed by gentle heat, and stained by Ziehl-Neelson's method, and examined for the presence of spermatozoa and smegma bacilli.

Presence of Microorganisms in the Uterus: The absence of sperms in the vagina does not mean that sexual intercourse has not taken place. It may be due to non-emission, aspermia, previous vasectomy, very old age, or poor technique by the examining doctor. Detection of seminal fluid from vasectomised males requires the demonstration of prostatic acid phosphatase which should be qualitatively distinguished from vaginal acid phosphatase by electrophoresis. Quantitatively, normal value of acid phosphatase in the vagina is 340 IU/litre. It rises to about 3000IU in about 2-3 hours after intercourse and gradually returns to normal in about 12-24 hours. Any level higher than 340 IU indicates seminal fluid. As a result of the discovery of semen specific glycoprotein (P30), acid phosphatase test is used only as a screening test. P30 is present in normal and aspermic semen. Graves et al found in some instances P30 test was positive when acid phosphatase test was negative. P30 is detectable in vaginal fluid for a mean period of 27 hours after intercourse as compared to 14 hours acid phosphatase. If semen is identified, determining of generic markers, if need be, can be done by enzyme studies and DNA typing. Swabbing of mouth, vagina, and anus for sperm detection should be performed on rape victims.

Sexually transmitted diseases (STDs): The disease for which the victims are at risk appear to be Chlamydial infection, Gonorrhea, Syphilis, Chancre, Genital wards ,Genital herpes, Trichomoniasis, Hepatitis B and HIV infection may be considered if the assailant appears to be so infected.

Collection of Laboratory Specimens: In some jurisdictions, sexual assault kits are provided by the law enforcing agency. They contain packing material, and instructions for collection and preservation of evidence that conform to standards laid down by the crime laboratory.

In those jurisdictions where no such kits are provided, it is necessary to consult the crime laboratory to ensure that the evidence meets with its requirements. The list of specimens to be collected from the victim for laboratory examination include:

Clothing-stained, torn, foreign matter Scrapings of dried blood stains-grouping, DNA characteristics Scrapings of dried seminal stains-grouping, sperms, P30 glycoprotein, DNA characteristics Hair-matted pubic hair, combed foreign hair, plucked hair Broken nails and debris from under the nails Blood- grouping, alcohol, drugs, VDRL, T cells Saliva-secretor status, and Swabs from any soiled area of skin; from the bite marks for saliva; and from mouth, pharynx, vagina, cervix, and anus for spermatozoa, microorganisms, P30 glycoprotein, and STD. other specimens, e.g. hair head, body hair, urine (for drugs, pregnancy), etc, are collected at the discretion of the examiner. The examination should be tailored to the requirement of the particular case and collection of all samples may not be necessary.

The Infernce: This depends very much upon circumstances. The site of offence may be examined if it appears desirable. In children, the examiner must not expect signs of struggle as they are normally not capable of exercising sufficient resistance to provoke injury. The superstitious belief that sexual intercourse with a virgin cures venereal disease has, on occasions, led to rape. Some girls are too terrified when an attack of rape is made upon them; they do not offer any resistance, with the result their bodies do not bear evidence of injuries as might be expected from a struggle, while locally there may be all the expected signs of accomplished act of penetration. In such a case, the acts and the "demeanour of the girl" (distressed, dazed, shocked, tearful, aggressive, etc) immediately after the alleged commission of crime should be subjected to very critical investigation, as these may provide valuable evidence, corroborative or otherwise, regarding the alleged ravishing. The mental condition and any signs of drunkenness should be particularly noted, if, on laboratory examination, a drug is found, the doctor should be prepared to state if the amount of drug is consistent with the degree of intoxication that would make valid consent improbable or impossible.

Follow-Up: The aim is to aid the victim to recover from the traumatic experience of sex assault and regain dignity and self-respect. According, follow-up involves treatment of injuries, tetanus prophylaxis, prevention and termination of pregnancy, prevention and treatment of any STD's and referral to crisis intervention centers for support by social workers and psychiatrists.

PHYSICAL EXAMINATION

1. Height
2. Weight
3. Breath; inspiration, expiration
4. Chest girth at the level of nipples
5. Abdominal girth at the level of navel
6. General built and appearance
7. Voice

8. Teeth
9. Hair: Axillary, pubic
10. Mammae-development of breast milk
11. Generative organs-development of genitals
12. Onset of puberty-date
13. Ossification report from radiological examination
14. Age
15. History
16. Date and hour when the female made complain and the precise words employed by her at the time, i.e. detailed account of the occurrence as given by the women.
17. General behavior
18. Date and the exact time when rape was said to have been committed
19. Place where it occurred
20. The exact circumstances under which the rape was committed i.e. whether the parties were standing or lying on the ground
21. Whether or not the female was menstruating at the time
22. Whether she was sensible during the whole time when the offence was committed or under any influence of alcohol, or other intoxicant
23. General feeling of those accompanying the female towards her and towards the accused
24. Whether she uttered any cries or was too terrified to do so
25. Clothing-if changed-when 26 Whether bath was taken-when
26. Whether urine was passed-when
27. Whether motion was passed-when
28. Mental condition and signs of drunkenness, if any
29. Gait
30. Intelligence
31. Demeanour
32. Examination of clothes including under-linen worn at the time of alleged rape and preserved for examination of blood, semen(including grouping if possible), other discharges Mud-dirt.
33. Injuries to cheeks, lips, mammae, thighs, and genitals
34. Genitals-pubic hair-length-matted or not; Vulva,vagina, Hymen, Fourchette, perineum, cervix
35. Is venereal disease present? Is there is a possibility of HIV transmission?
36. Smears From vagina, for spermatozoa and microorganisms from urethra for gonorrhea, from sore for evidence of syphilis or chancroid
37. Blood group examination if consent available

38. Other examination, e.g. for pregnancy, HIV infection
39. Date, Signature of the Medical Officer with designation

UNNATURAL SEXUAL OFFENCES

SODOMY

The practice of sodomy was said to be common in town, mentioned in the bible, by the name "SODOM" from which the word sodomy is derived.[1]

The anal coitus is also known as GREEK LOVE or sin of Sodom.

In modern practice sodomy means anal intercourse between two males (homosexual sodomy) or between a male and female it is known as (heterosexual sodomy) it is also called "buggery".[1,2,3,4,5,6]

It is termed "gerontophilia" when the passive agent is an adult, and "paederasty", when the passive agent is a young boy and the boy is called "catamite". The active agent is one who performs the act and the passive agent is one on whom the act is performed.[1-6]

The one who practice is known as "sodomite".[1]

A pedophile is an adult who repeatedly engages in sexual activities with children below the age of puberty. Opinion as to cause of the dilatation should be guarded and it should only be stated that it is consistent with entry of a penis. The consent of sodomy is of no value, as both partners are punishable.[2] The only proof of sodomy is presence of semen in the anus.[1,2,3,4,5,6]

It is necessary that penetration, however little, should be proved strictly in order that offences of sodomy are made punishable under section 377 IPC.

An attempt to commit this offence is punishable under section 511 IPC, with imprisonment for life or other imprisonment.[2,3,4,5]

SODOMY may be performed by two men who alternatively act as active and passive agent. The question of consent does not arise and it is no defence that the passive partly was the accuser's wife. Both offenders are punishable under section 377 IPC, but when the offences is done without the consent of the passive agent, the active agent alone is guilty.[1]

Homosexual practice is common in all classes of society. The offence is common among prisoners, members of armed forces, and sailors, who are sex- starvated by circumstances. The act is difficult to perform against the will unless the person is drugged or drunk.[1,6]

In some parts of India there is a class of male prostitutes commonly known as "Eunuchs" and Hizras act as passive agent. Zenanas (male transvestites), with intact male gentiles but dressed like female part and dress their hair in female fashion , wear ornaments and adopt tastes and habit like female , may act as both active and passive agents.[2,3,4,6]

The two groups live separately and preserve a line of demarcation between them.

A group of 47 Lucknow eunuchs were studied in details by. K. B. Kunwar. Most of these have a compulsive urge to homosexuality but there are few whoa are latent homosexuals andsome who indulges occasionally with an exploratory sense or when they are deprived of contact with the members of opposite sex.[4]

According to Kinsey 4% of Americans are exclusively homosexuals while Desmond Currans and Denis Parr found 5 in series of private patients. A homosexual component exist in everybody, so in the sense it is universal, but it varies quantitatively in different individuals and also varies at different epochs in life. The condition is one of arrested development or natural deviation and beyond that homosexuality is a diseases. It exist among all calling and at all levels of society. A prison sentence may do more harm than good, psychotherapy is useful in some.

In few cases that come for trial before a court of law, the active agent is usually a grownup male child, the passive agent, a boy and occasionally a girl or woman.

For the investigation of this offences medical examiner, are also applicable and active agent is necessary as in the case of rape. It must be necessary to inquire if the activity agent had obtained the consent of that passive agent for this purpose by means of physical force or fraud, or of the active agent y the reason of age or diseases, was physically unfit t commit the offence. A grown up passive agent may persuade a young boy to act as an active agent to practise the vice on him, but such instances are very rare indeed. Modi had seen only one case in which a passive agent of 45 to 50 years of age was prosecuted for having persuaded a boy of 16 years to commit unnatural connection with him. In false accusations modi had often heard a story that the accused was sleeping in the same bed with the victim , and he committed the unnatural offence on the later while he was asleep. It should be borne in mind that it is not possible for an adult male to accomplish the act on a boy during sleep without awaking him on another healthy male against his will. [4]

Such cases are usually examined on request from investigating police officer following on order from judicial magistrate court. Some times a child with severe injuries around anal orifices may be brought by parents directly to Hospital. Attending doctors must examine and provide treatment to the child and send injury report to local police station. [3,4]

Marriage is taken as an implied consent by the wife for normal intercourse anal not for anal intercourse. If the wife consented both are guilty; if she did not, the husband alone is guilty. Under section 13 of Hindu Marriage Act 1995, a wife can apply for annulment of marriage if husband has been guilty of rape, sodomy or bestiality.

In England the sexual offences Act 1967 provides hat it shall not be an offence for man to commit buggery or gross indecency with another man provided that act is carried out in private between consenting parties, each of whom is above the age of 21 years. [4]

For the investigation of the crime, a medical examination of both passive and active agent is necessary It should be remembered that false charges may be made for purposes of blackmail and en be tricked into homosexual relationship by men masquerading as women whilst on shore, particularly in eastern seas. [1]

EXAMINATION OF THE VICTIM

- ❖ Consent should be taken before examination.
- ❖ History is taken as regards to sites of injuries and behavioural characteristics of assailant
- ❖ The victim is examined in the knee elbow position with proper lighting.
- ❖ Presence of 3rd position is also needed. [2]

EXAMINATION OF THE ACTIVE AGENT OF THE SODOM

Pre-requisites and preliminary particles

- General information – name, sex, age , address, occupation, time , date, and place of the examination
- Two identification marks are noted.
- Consent in this case is guided.

- History, date, time of the incident defecation, change of clothing, bathing, washing the anal area after the alleged act, use of lubricant and degree of penetration is specifically asked for.
- Any history of pain/ burning sensation associated with defecation walking is specifically asked for.
- Gait of the victim is noted.

SIGN OF SODOMY ON EXAMINATION OF ACTIVE AGENT

- This is almost similar to that found in male accused of rape case.
- The accused should be examined for abrasions and bruises on the glans
- or tearing of the fraenum of the penis, for the traces of faeces and lubricant about his genitals, and for the peculiar smell transferred by the glans .
- Faecal soiling, blood and foreign hairs are most likely to become trapped in the area of coronal sulcus particularly in the uncircumcised.
- His clothes should be examined for the presence of stain either seminal, faecal, blood or mud and his body for marks of struggle. In addition, any evidence of venereal diseases should look for.
- If there is no great disproportion between the size of the anus and that of the penis, it is highly improbable that any sign will be found.
- In a habitual active gent, there may be elongation and constriction of the penis with cons sequent angulations of the urethra, on account of the constricting force of the sphincter ani. [1,3,6]

MEDICO LEGAL ASPECT

- Presently, if the act is done, without the consent of the adult passive partner, the active partner is held guilty; otherwise it is not consideredas an offence.
- Marriage contract gives implied consent for sexual intercourse per vaginum, not per anum. Under section 13 of Hindu Marriage Act, conviction for natural or unnatural sexual act is a valid ground for divorce.
- Penetrative anal sex is legal in UK between consenting adults who are over the age of consent, i.e. at least 16 years of age. The sexual act had to take place in private and members of the Armed Forces and merchant seamen were excluded whatever their age.

Pre- Requisites and Preliminary Particulars:

- Written authorization from Magistrate or in charge of the police station is a must before undertaking an examination . if the passive agent is a victim (non- consenting) he can also request for an examination, but the doctor should inform the police.
- General information – name, sex, age , address, occupation, time , date, and place of the examination

- Two identification marks are noted.
- Consent in this case is guided.
- History, date, time of the incident defecation, change of clothing, bathing, washing the anal area after the alleged act, use of lubricant and degree of penetration is specifically asked for.
- Any history of pain/ burning sensation associated with defecation walking is specifically asked for.
- Gait of the victim is noted[1]

CLOTHING - are examined for damage, loose pubic hair, stains of blood /semen/ lubricant faeces.

SIGN OF SODOMY ON EXAMINTAION OF PASSIVE AGENT

In a recent offences (not habituated)

- Lesions are marked in children because of great disproportion in size between the orifice of the victim and penis of the accused. A perianal and rectal swab should be taken first and any matted (anal/pubic) or foreign hair should be preserved for examination.
- There is pain/ tenderness during examination.
- Smears of lubricant and loose foreign pubic hair around / in the anus.
- Fresh /dried semen may be present around / in the anus[6]
- Signs of struggle (nail scratch abrasion, bruise, teeth bite marks etc.) if done without consent.
- Stains of lubricant jelly blood or semen or both in about the anus and clothing's.
- Bruises, abrasions, excoriations, or slight laceration of the anal mucous membrane may be found, especially if the passive agent is a young boy unaccustomed to such acts before.
- There may be anal prolapse[6]
- Digital examination is painful , may show loss of elasticity and tone.6
- Characteristic gonorrhoeal discharge on cloth or near about the anus, if the active agent is suffering from the disease.[1,2,3,5,6]

The examination should be carried out in **knee – elbow** position, and n presence of a third person. In most charges of sodomy the victim is boy or young man.[1,2,3,4,5,6]

A number of variables may affect the possibility of finding evidence.

- Frequents of the acts.
- Time interval between intercourse and examination.
- Age, built and size of the orifice in the individual.

285

- Degree of force applied during the act.
- Size of penile organ.
- Cooperativeness of the partner.
- Use of lubricants[6]

If he is not accustomed to sodomy, the following signs may be found.[1]

GENITALS SIGNS-

- Anal orifice is found dilated, irritable, and tender to touch, a zone of bruising may be seen around the orifice.
- There are often slight abrasions may be seen between the anus and the tip of coccyx.
- If there is gradual but forcible out stretching, a radial fissure of the mucous membrane of the anus will be found.
- If sudden violence is used, there is often a triangular bruised tear of the posterior part of the anus with its base external .
- Anal and perianal swabs should be taken for examination of spermatozoa, evidence of venereal infection ad presence of lubricant . a sample of hair preferably any matted hair, should also be taken.
- The anal canal and lower rectum should then be carefully be inspected through a proctoscope and any area of injury or abnormality of the mucosal lining must be noted.
- The person may complain of pain when the anal canal is being examined.
- gait and defecation may also be painful.[1,4,5,6]

OTHER SIGNS-

- Additional evidence may be found e.g. Presence of spermatozoa on the clothing and signs of struggle.
- The clothing should in all cases be subjected to laboratory examination for the presence of stains either seminal ,faecal, blood or mud.
- The only evidence of sodomy is the presence of semen in the anus. Any option as to the cause of dilatation should be guarded , merely state that it is consistent with the entry of a penis.[1,2,3,4,6]

SIGNS AND EXAMMNATION OF HABITUAL SODOMIST

- If the victim is a habitual sodomist, he lies in the knee elbow position , with prolapsed mucous membrane from anal canal.
- Funnel shaped anus with thickening and smoothing of anal skin.
- Perianal hairs are often found shaved.
- Loss of rugosity of the anal mucous membrane
- Loss of tonocity of the sphincter ani.
- Excoriation and cicatrisation of the old ulcers or abrasions in and around the anus.
- Ill or undeveloped genital organs.
- Signs of the implanted or venereal diseases are strong corroborative evidence. Age of the passive agents must also be ascertained for criminal responsibility.
- There may be old healed scars from previous stretching and splitting.
- There may be feminine gait and manner of speaking.
- Loss of usual mucosal fold, i.e. smooth mucous membrane.
- The presence of a fissure or fissure scar is not uncommon and external and internal haemorrhoids may be present.
- Anus dilated with keratinisation of the mucosa.
- Anal hairs may be shaved but not be necessary the pubic hairs.
- Person does not experience any pain or tenderness during digital examination. Anal sphincter is lax, opening is patulous, canal is dilated and there may be loss of fine symmetrical rugal pattern along with congested or dilated viens.[6]
- Lateral traction- external anal sphincter relaxes reflexly when biannual traction is applied to the buttocks.[6]
- Anal opening- is more deep situated than usual due to absorption of subcutaneous fat, giving a funnel shaped depression of buttocks.[6]

Homosexuals commonly exhibit feminine traits as regards dress, cosmetics, gait, and manner of speaking.

Sometimes a child may be thrilled to suppress that anal coitus was performed on him. [1,2,3,4,5,6]

PASSIVE AGENT	ACTIVE AGENT
• Clothing • Swab for anal canal • Swab for bite mark • Blood • Nail scraping • Matted and foreign pubic hair and his own for comparison	• Clothing • Swab for glans • Urethral • Blood • Pubic hair • Nail scraping • Urine

SIGNS OF UNWILLING PARTNER

- Parts around the anus are usually tender due to bruising of the anal margins with splitting of the skin or tearing of lining within the rectum and stretching of the anus it self .
- Examination of the passive partner should include swabs for seminal fluid and lubricants. Foreign hairs should be collected.[2]

EXAMINATION OF ASSAILANT (ACTIVE SODOMY)

Assailant is examined for his age, mental condition and signs of resistance, bloodstains and venereal diseases. Victim blood hair or faecal stain may be found an assailant clothes or private parts. Proforma for examination is enclose. [2]

DIFFICULTY IN DIAGNOSIS

Examination of alleged sexual offences between males and presents rather more difficulty to the inexperienced doctor. In fact it is not surprising that many pathologists who have not examined anal orifice in life are misled by the appearances after when the sphincter is relaxed. An extremely difficult examination is in connection with divorce when woman alleges abnormal practices against the husband. The anal orifice can be quite lax following child birth, particularly if there has been a perineal tear, some healed fissure and old haemorrhoids may be a normal finding making it extremely difficult to say for certain weather the allegation is true unless it has been persistent practice such practice is not uncommon.[1]

BESTALITY/ (ZOOPHILIA)

This means sexual intercourse human being with pet or domestic animal, lower animal by a male or a female such intercourse are usually done through the anus and vagina and involvement of those animals which are tamed such as she-goat she-ass cow-duck etc. and are kept on farm or as pets example-donkey, pig, goat, cattle, chicken ,dog, cat or in households.[1,2,3,4,5,6]

Vaginal intercourse is most common.[2]

In such cases fluid from vagina of the animal and that the discharge adhering to the surrounding hairs on its genitals should be examined for human seminal fluid and spermatozoa. The presence of this is a positive approve of the offence.[3]

This offence is punishable under section 377 IPC.[1,2,3,4,5,6]

- ❖ The hair of the animal may also be found on the pubic area of the accused or on his cloth.[1,3,4,5,6]
- ❖ Sometimes injuries caused by kicks of animal e.g.- cow, buffalo, donkey may be seen over the person of male accused.[1,3,4,6]
- ❖ Rarely a female subject may be charged committing this offence with male pet animals.[3]
- ❖ It is most commonly seen person suffering from mental abnormalities.[1,2,3]
- ❖ On most occasions, the animal manipulates the genitalia by mouth and actual coitus is not quite common.[1,2,3,5]

It is a sexual intercourse with animal, either vaginal, anal or oral. This includes all animals, including birds, the usual victim being pets and farm animals[6]

- ❖ Generally , sheep are used by male, and dogs or cats ye females as they are easily available and relative docile.[1,3,6]
- ❖ Doctors may sometimes be asked to examine genital injuries or infections in a man acquired during such episodes.[1,4,6]
- ❖ The sure evidence of bestiality is finding of human spermatozoa the genital tract of the animal.[1,2,3,4,5,6]
- ❖ The penis may be contaminated with faecal matter, vaginal secretion or hair of the animal. There may be injury to the penis , dung stains , generally body injuries due to the kicks and some blood stains. [1,6]

Sexual intercourse usually takes place through the vagina, but it may take place through the anus or any other orifice fit to receive the male genital organ.[4]

- ❖ In one case sexual intercourse per nose with bullock was regarded as a case of bestiality with in the terms of section 377 IPC.[4]
- ❖ In UK, under SEXUAL OFFENCES ACT 2003 reduced the sentence to a maximum of 2 years imprisonment for penile of or by an animal.

The lower animals that are selected for this purpose are cows, mares, she-asses, goats, itches and even hens.

Cases of bestiality, through rare, do occur among young and vigorous villagers who go out to graze cattle's in fields far away from the gays of human eye.[1,4]

Owing to loneliness and proximity of animals they are exited to commit this abdominal crime.

The accused may be young person employed to look after the animals, sex-starved lonely individual or some of these men have mental abnormalities. [1,2,4]

The crime of bestiality is also seen in some ignorant men, who have superstitious believes that they are cured for gonorrhoea by committing sexual intercourse with a she-ass. [1,4]

The crime may be committed with any animal, provided that intercourse, whether per annum or per vaginum is physically possible.

In one English case it was hold that an accused could not be found guilty of bestiality with a domestic foul whose parts where to small to admit those of the accused which were torn away in the attempt.

In a subsequent case it was held that a person could be found guilty of attempt to commit the offence with a duck, presumably on the principle that it is punishable to attempt to commit a criminal act which infact is impossible of accomplishment.

A person who can be convicted of aiding and abetting an innocent person to commit bestiality. In R.V.v Bourne [1952] a man sexually excited a dog compelled his wife to submit to a connection with the dog, for which he was convicted of aiding and abetting his wife to commit bestiality.

In such cases of bestiality the perpetrators of the crime are caught red handed; medical evidence, therefore is not required to prove the offence. But, as false accusation by the village chaukidars and others are not uncommon in India.

It is necessary that both the accused an animal alleged to have been used for the purpose should be examined by a medical officer.

❖ The only important sign confirming the commission of the crime are the presence human spermatozoa in the vaginal or the anal canal of the animal,
❖ The presence of the human hairs especially of its external genitals, on the person or the clothing of the accused together with some suspicious stains of the dung or blood or abrasion on his generative organs.
❖ In addition there may be the marks of injury on the person of the accused caused by kicks teeth or claws of the animal.
❖ Sometimes, laceration on the anus or external genitals of the passive animal with effusion blood may be found.
❖ The presence of gonorrhoeal discharge in the vagina of an animal,
❖ Especially a she-ass is a positive sign of bestiality as gonorrhoea does not occur naturally in such animal.
❖ Among half a dozen cases of bestiality reported by Modi in Agra during a period of 11 years modi could give a definite opinion only in one case from identifying by microscopic examinations the hairs of passive animal found under the prepuce , on the thighs on the loin cloth [dhoti of the accused].[4]

Sure evidence – of bestiality is finding of human spermatozoa in the genital tract of the animal and animal hair on the onside of the pant or under the prepuce (Locard's principleof exchange). Both the accused as well as the animal should be examined.

Finding on the accused- the penis may be contaminated by the faecal matter, vaginal secretion, or hair of the animal.

There may be injury to penis if such intercourse is through anus.

Dung stains , animals hairs and injuries due to kicks, teeth or claws of the animal may be found on the clothes and on the body of accused. In the event.1,6

The animal is injured during the act, and is as a result therefore, there are blood stains on the clothes or on the body of accused, important evidence may be obtained by establishing species of blood stains by the precipitin test.[1,6]

Finding on the animal-

- ❖ Human spermatozoa may be present in the vagina or anus of the animal
- ❖ The spermatozoa of lower animals can be differentiated from those of microscopically.[1,3,5]
- ❖ Sometimes, human hair may be found sticking to the animal.
- ❖ Human hair can be differenced from animal hair by microscopic examination.
- ❖ Injuries may be found on the orifice of animal.
- ❖ The presence of gonorrhoeal discharge in the vagina of an animal is a positive sign of bestiality as gonorrhoea does not naturally occur in animals.[1,3,4,5,6]
- ❖ Examination by a veterinary surgeon is helpful.[1]

TRIBADISM / LESBIANISM

This means sexual connection between two females [prevalent in island of lesbos]. It is a form of mental aberration.[1,3,4,5]

It is also known as lesbian love or lesbianism. [1,2,3,4,5,6]

The word "tribadism" is derived from the obsolete word tribade, meaning "lesbian".[6]

According to Greek mythology, the female population of isle of lesbos practiced this perversion and hence the name. it is also known as female homosexuality/ lesbian. [1,3]

The term has to have its current meaning due to ancient GREEK poet, Sappho, who lives on the island ; some of her poem are concerned love between n women. This led to the term sapphism being used lesbianism.[6]

Homosexuality_– it is the phenomenon where in an individual (Male or Female) prefers a partner of the sae sex, for sexual activity and intimae bonding.

- ❖ The most frequent form of male homosexual activity is fellatio and masturbation; anal intercourse occurs much less often.
- ❖ In the past, homosexual couples often lived together but downplayed their relationship in public to avoid discrimination. Many couples now asse the legitimacy of this relationship though marriage (recognised by religious and political institutions) and parent hood.
- ❖ Lesbians couples are conceiving and bearing children through various artificial methods like infertile heterosexual couples. Adoption is another means to parenthood for gay and lesbian couples.

Homosexuality means persistent emotional and physical attraction to members of same sex. Female homosexuality is known as tribalism or lesbianism. Sexual gratification of women is obtained by other women by simple lip kissing, generalised body contact, deep kissing , manipulation of breast and genitalia , genitals opposition friction of genital external organs.[2,6]

Gratification means sexual desire of women by another women[1]

- The instrument of passion is usually the clitoris which may be enlarged or artificial penis or phallus may be used.[1,2,3,4,5,6]
- The predominant form of sexual activity to achieve orgasm are oral genital and manual genital stimulation. Self stimulation of clitoris is frequently the preferred method.[6]

Many lesbians are masculine in type possibly because of endocrine disturbances.[2,4,5,6]

Aristophanes mention the use of an artificial penis or phallus by melesian females. This sort of sexual inversion is found among such women though such cases have been rarely brought before a court of law and this is not covered by section 377 IPC.[4]

Such homosexual women are in different towards men.[3,4]

External genitilia of these women may show;

- Scratch marks abrasions.
- Teeth marks.[2,3,4,5,6]

Question of penetration of vulva of the passion women does not rise.[3]

- A lesbian may commit suicide or murder of her partner when her partner marries or get engaged with a male subject.[1,2,3,4,6]
- Due to endocrine disturbances such women are usually mentally defective or who suffer from nymphomania [excessive sexual desire] and hate opposite sex [male].[1,2,4,6]
- Lesbians who are jealous of one another , when rejected may commit suicide of homicide or both.[2,4,6]
- Tribalism is usually indulged in by women who have repulsion for men or who suffers from perverted uncontrollable sexual desire [nymphomania].
- The condition is of little medico legal interest and medical examination is of no value in deciding whether the offence has taken place. [1,2,3,4,5]

In a case where a husband petitioned for divorce on the ground of his wife cruelty the judge held that a wife's unnatural relations with another women , coupled with neglect of her husband and home which so prayed upon the husbands health that it broke down, constituted a course of conduct which not only injured the health but gave rise to reasonable apprehension of future injury therefore the husband was entitled to a decree.

Homosexual women are generally mental degenerates, and have often natural antipathy in difference towards individuals of the opposite sex. On the other hand, the are so morbidly jealous of the women with whom they are in inverted love that they are sometimes incited to commit even murder. [4,6]

Buccal coitus(Sin of Gomorrah)

Buccal coitus or intercourse per os also falls under section 377IPC and is punishable accordingly.[1,2,4,6]

Intercourse through the mouth is usually practiced by adult males on children. It is called sin of Gomorrah because but is prevalent in Biblical town of that name. [1,4,6]

It denotes penile or vaginal oral sexual intercourse and can be performed by both males and females.[6]

Due to introducing the male organ in the mouth of a young child. Sudden accidental death from asphyxia may occur from aspiration of semen or impaction of penis in the lower part of pharynx.

In such suspicious smears from trachea should be examined for sperms and acid phosphates. It is practiced mainly by prostitutes.

Male prostitutes are called **eunuchs,** castrated eunuchs are called **hijrahs** and eunuchs with intact genitalia are known as Zenana.[2]

Buccal swabs from the victim within about 8 hours of oral penile contact, provided there has been no clearing of teeth nor consumption of hot drinks, will frequently reveal seminal traces. Rarely, faint teeth marks and abrasions may be seen on the penis of assailant.

Fellatio means the oral stimulation or manipulation of the penis by either the male or female.

Cunnilingus means the oral stimulation of then female genitals[.1]

Buccal coitus, sometimes a male accused may be introduced erect penis in the mouth of a male or female child.

Detection of abrasion and superficial laceration on the penis and detection of seminal fluid from oral and pharyngeal swab of victim will prove the offence [3,5]

Coitus as per os(the sin of Gomorrah) falls within the provision of and is punishable under section 377IPC.

The sin of Gomorrah is punishable in a case, in which one Khanu was found guilty under the section of 377 I.P.C of having committed the sin of Gomorrah (Coitus as per os) wuth a certain little child, the innocent accomplice of his abomination Kennedy , J .C ., observed that " there is no intercourse unless the visiting member is enveloped , at least partly by the visited organisms, for intercourse connotes reciprocity, looking at, the question in this way it would seem that sin of Gomorrah is no less carnal intercourse that the sin of Sodom." [4]

Buccal coitus denotes penile or vaginal oral sexual intercourse and can be performed by both males and females.

- It is also called as sin of Gomorrah , because it is alleged that buccal coitus was prevalent in Gomorrah , the biblical twin of Sodom.
- Fellatio (Latin fellare: to suck) means oral stimulation of penis either by male or female.
- Cunnilingus means oral stimulation of female genitalia.
- Earlier buccal coitus was considered as a sexual deviation, but nowadays it is considered normal sexual foreplay.
- Anilingus- the practice of oral stimulation of the anus.
- Urningism-sexual practice in which sexual desire is only for one of the same sex (obsolete word for male homosexuality [6]

Injuries- A person who is forced to perform fellatio may have trauma in the oral cavity, such as petechiae of the palate and/ or posterior pharynx.

Tears to the liable frenulum may result from forceful traction on th upper lip. If a fellator's scalp hair is grasped forcibily during the act, traction alopecia may be seen.

- If the victim has fellatio or cunnilingus performed on him or her , acute sign include petechiae, abrasions or bite marks to the genitalia.
- The only material evidence of buccal coitus is the presence of seminal products including spermatozoa in oral cavity and nasopharynx of the

fellator (dependent upon time since contact and history of ejaculation) and buccal mucosal cells on the external genitalia of the subject.

- The mouth and the pharynx should be swabbed with non absorbent cotton swabs and smear should make similar to that made of vaginal material. A culture for gonorrhoea should be taken form nasophayrnx.

MEDICOLEGAL ASPECT

- In India, the Hindu Marriage Act, insistence on buccal coitus , if it is non- consensual and repetitive , constitutes a valid ground for divorce.
- Buccal coitus performed by consenting adults over 21 years of age is permitted by law in UK.[6]

DELHI HIGHCOURT RULING ON SECTION 377 IPC

Delhi high court alloying a petition and observed that "we declare that section 377 IPC , in so far it criminalises consensual sexual acts of adults in private, is violative of articles 21, 14 and 15 of the constitution.

The provisions of section 377 IPC will continue to govern non consensual penile non vaginal sex and penile non vaginal sex involving minors. By "adult" we mean everyone who is 18 years of age and above.

A person below 18 would be presumed not to be able to consent to a sexual act. This clarification will hold till , of course , parliament chooses amend the law to effectuate the recommendation of the law commission of India in its 172nd report, which we believe removes a great deal of confusion.

Secondly, we clarify that are judgement will not result in re opening of criminal cases involving section 377 IPC that have already attained finality. [Para 132,Naz Foundation v/s Government of NCT of Delhi and Others , WP [C] no. 7455/2001, date discussion ; 2nd July , 2009]. However, this was set aside justice SJ Mukerjee and GS Singhvi of honourable supreme court of India in the judgement dated 11 December, 2013 and hold that "we hold that section 377 IPC does not suffer from the vice of unconstutionality of the declaration made by the decision bench of high court is legally unsustainable". So for now the section 377 IPC is a punishable offence whether consensual or not and is liable for punishment as we mentioned before. [2]

SECTION 377- unnatural sexual offences: who ever voluntary has carnal intercourse against the order of nature with nay man, woman or animal, shall be punished with imprisonment for life, or with imprisonment of either description for term which may extend to 10 years, and shall also be liable to fine.

EXPLANATION- penetration is sufficient to constitute the carnal intercourse, necessary to the offence described in this section.

IPC377- criminalizes any penetration sex that does not lead to reproduction\, thereby criminalizing sexual expression by homosexuals, bisexuals and trans-sexual.[2]

Classification of offence- imprisonment for the life .

Imprisonment for 10 years and fine –cognizable – non baiable- Triable by magistrate of first class non – compoundable.

Sexually Transmitted Diseases

STD'S – the diseases for which the victim is at risk to be appear to be –

- **a-** Chlamydial infection
- **b-** gonorrhoea
- **c-** syphilis
- **d-** chancre
- **e-** genital warts
- **f-** genital herpes,
- **g-** trichomoniasis

Hepatits B and HIV infection may be considered if the assailant appears to be infected.

Chlamydial infection is common. Its prophylaxis is the same a s that for gonorrhoea.

Trichominiasis, genital wart, and herpes are not common. They need to be considered if symptoms arise. Most authors therefore suggest a cervical culture for gonorrhoea and Chlamydia (if laboratory facilities are available), and a blood test for syphilis , and other test are required. The following procedure is recommended.

The presence or absence of any urethral or vaginal discharge should be noted. it may be due to gonorrhoea, vaginitis worms, or uncleanliness. The presence or sores should be looked for. They may be due to syphilis or chancroid blood should be examined for T – cells if there is suspicious of transmission of HIV. A substantial drop of T cell count at the end of 3 weeks is serious warning and need further investigation.

In gonorrhoea, a purulent discharge is generally seen after three days. A thin film of discharge is made on two three glass sides, fixed and stained by Gram 's Method, and examined under the high power of microscope. Gonococci when present, are seen in intracellular, Gram negative , bean shaped diplococci. In case of negative result , an opinion can be given only after three consecutive examinations have been made at intervals of one week each. A negative smear at the time of examination may be pf significance if positive smear at the time of examination may be of significance if possible smear is obtained within a few days of assault.

If oral or rectal contact has occurred, specimen for gonorrhoea culture needs to be taken from the mouth, pharynx and tonsillar area or the rectum.

If there is a sore which is suspected to be syphilitic, the discharge is examined under dark ground illumination for the presence of treponema palladium. Blood for serological test (VDRL) is also collected. An initial negative result followed by positive result at six weeks or later is of value.

If the sore is suspected to be due to chancroid , the smear made from the discharge or bubo fluid when stained by Gram method will show the presence of Ducrey's bacillus. It is a Gram Negative streptobacillus with rounded ends.

The STD's can be attributed to the accused only when

 i- The accused is also suffering from the venereal disease.

ii- the disease appeared in the victim after its known period of incubation after the alleged sexual assault,

iii- the victim was not suffering from the disease prior to this assault.

The incubation period of gonorrhoea is 2-8 days . it may vary from 1-15 days.

The incubation period of syphilis is 2-8 weeks . the average being 25days the incubation period of chancriod varies from 3 weeks to 3 months.

REFERENCES

1. Parikh C. K., Parikh's textbook of medical jurisprudence forensic and toxicology, 6th edition (2011), C.B.S. Publishers and Distributors, Ansari Road, Darya Ganj , New Delhi (p.5.50-5.30)
2. Mahanta Putul , Modern Textbook of Forensic Medicine And Toxiocology (2014) , Jaypee Brothers Medical Publishers , Darya Ganj , New Delhi.(p.412,433- 434)
3. A. K. Gupta, Essentials of Forensic Medicine and Toxicology, 5th edition (2014) Current Books International , 60, Lenin, Saranee, Kolkata – 700013.(p.178- 180)
4. Modi, Jaising P Textbook of Medical Jurisprudence And Toxicology 21th edition (1997) N M Tripathi Limited , Bombay.(p. 360-353)
5. Basu S.C . Handbook of forensic Medicine And Toxicology, 3rd edition(2007), Current Distributors, Lenin Saranee, Calcutta, (p. 127, 128)
6. Gautam Biswas , Review of Forensic Medicine and Toxoicology , 2nd edition (2014), Jaypee Brothers Medical Publishers P Ltd, 4838/24 Ansari Road, Darya Ganj, New Delhi -110002. (p. 340- 343)
7. Usmani Hammad, Tib- ul – Qanoon, 1st edition (1976), Universal Book House, Allahbad. (p.296-298)
8. www.Wikipedia.com

Book Details

Author: Izharul H.
Book Title: Essential textbook of medical jurisprudence
Paperback: 299 pages
Publisher: CS Independent Publishing Platform; 1 edition (November 28, 2014)
Language: English
ISBN-10: **1508841934**
ISBN-13: **978-1508841937**
Product Dimensions: 7 x 10 inches

Other Books of the author:

Essential Textbook of Preventive and Social Medicine

Humoral Pathology: Adjustment and Regulation

Essential Hand Book of Toxicology: For Medical Undergraduates

A Textbook of Regimenal Therapy: ...an unani speciality

Encyclopedia of Home Remedies to get Healthy Life

The Prime: MCQs for Post Graduation Unani Entrance Examination

The Premier, Previous Examination Papers Of MD Unani AMU Aligarh

www.ingramcontent.com/pod-product-compliance
Lightning Source LLC
Chambersburg PA
CBHW080759180526
45168CB00006B/2269